The Easy Steps to a Sane Body Through a Healthy Mouth

A Healthier Lifestyle

Karah Viniz

losses, direct or indirect, that are incurred as a result of the use of the information contained within this document, including, but not limited to, errors, omissions, or inaccuracies.

Table Of Contents

Introduction

A healthy smile is a reflection of a healthy mind and a healthy body. — Dr. Manasi Baweja.

Among all the beautiful blessings of life, a smile is a miraculous way of conveying various gestures. Each one of us aspires to visualize and feel immense pleasure and happiness in one's life, but this is possible only when a person is hail and healthy in every aspect of their life, whether it be physical, psychological, or oral. In the haste of life, we manage to keep up with our physical and mental wellness. However, most of us overlook the most important aspect of health, which is oral health. Mouth health is not confined to maintaining strong and healthy teeth, gums, and oral cavities. Instead, it is directly or indirectly associated with our overall health and body metabolism in some or other ways. To achieve this ultimate goal of a healthy mouth and sane body, one must explore the ABCs of oral hygiene and habits that form the key to moving ahead in this journey. Apart from this, it is also crucial to identify and choose the best prerequisites that are a must for one to aim for a healthy and bright smile with strong teeth.

It is difficult or almost impossible for us to get started with the endeavor to attain dental goals unless we know and understand how a good and healthy mouth can be a life changer. Along with retaining the longevity of teeth, good oral health also supports minimizing the chances of falling prey to various chronic diseases. Moreover, it boosts our self-confidence by bestowing us with a beautiful smile, enhancing our personality, and providing overall wellness. On the whole, maintaining good dental health saves money and time by reducing the number of dental visits. Apart from this, it is also necessary for us to have awareness and complete knowledge about the red flags that indicate the early warning signs and symptoms of any arising dental issue. Some of the most observed symptoms that must never be ignored are swollen and bleeding gums, cracked teeth, sensitivity and pain in teeth, dry mouth, and mouth ulcers. Furthermore, many critical health conditions tend to aggravate the complications of oral health issues. For instance, people who are suffering from diabetes, heart disease, or respiratory disorders are at a higher risk of developing oral comorbidities like gingivitis, tooth decay, cavities, or periodontitis.

The journey of striving for a confident smile and healthy mouth is often accompanied by various unseen and unexpected barriers and problems that may demoralize and deviate one from reaching their ultimate goal. Various unhealthy practices like improper eating, addictions, lack of awareness, and inability to maintain proper oral hygiene become the major pitfalls that restrict one from focusing on their overall wellness. Thus, to find a way out of this darkness, we must get equipped with various quick tips and hacks to improve our oral health. Some simple ways we can adopt to find visible change in our lives are regularly brushing our teeth, quitting unhealthy habits like smoking cigarettes and drinking alcohol and visiting the dentist regularly. Apart from this, cleaning the tongue, flossing teeth, using mouthwash, and changing the toothbrush regularly can be easily implemented to contribute toward a positive change in our oral health.

Maintaining good dental health can be an interesting and engaging task if we dive deeper into dentistry and explore the mind-boggling facts and unbelievable myths related to oral health. There are innumerable facts that might leave you stunned and speechless if you uncover them individually. Apart from this, it is necessary to get introduced to the fallacies that surround oral health in order to gain awareness and prevent any mistakes while moving ahead in the journey of attaining a healthy smile. Furthermore, the endeavor to achieve a healthy mouth and a sane body is impossible without assessing and self-examining one's oral health by finding answers to innumerable intriguing questions that are directly or indirectly related to our oral and overall wellness. Now, the wait is over, and here we present to you the best guide and mentor to direct you toward reaching the goal of achieving ultimate oral wellness in an elaborate and stepwise manner. It's a time when your mind would be occupied with various questions that might puzzle you. So, let's dive deep into this mesmerizing world to explore, understand, and learn how to achieve a healthy mouth and sane body.

Chapter 1:

Exploring the ABCs of

Oral Health

When you take care of your teeth, every word you speak, and every smile you share becomes a testament to your health. — Dr. Farrah Alsoudi, DDS

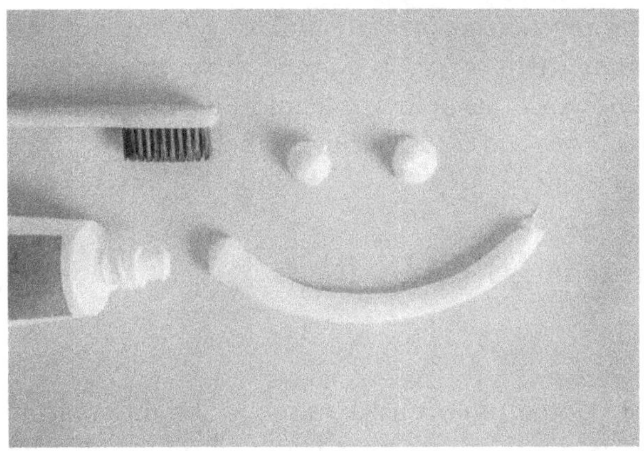

In the hustle and bustle of today's busy world, maintaining good oral health is one such issue that does not seem to intrigue the attention of many of us unless we get into any sort of serious issue. Many assume that maintaining a healthy mouth is simply confined to brushing our teeth regularly, using mouthwash, and flossing our teeth after every meal. However, the fact is that our oral health is influenced by many more interesting factors that directly or indirectly impact our overall wellness and quality of lifestyle. Scientific researchers advocate adopting various healthy practices like eating a nutritious and balanced diet, following healthy oral hygiene habits, staying away from smoking and drinking, and the list is too long.

Furthermore, a less-known fact is that oral health positively contributes toward improving our physical and mental wellness by slowing down aging, boosting immunity, and enhancing body metabolism. But, without an in-depth understanding of how valuable our oral health is, we can never make the required efforts to improve it for our long-term benefit. So, let's start the interesting journey toward finding genuine answers to the important what, why, and how related to oral health, which instantly come into our minds as we aim to achieve good oral hygiene and health goals.

What is Oral Health?

Most people often mistake a good, bright smile for a healthy mouth. However, a beautiful smile only adds to the beauty, boosts confidence, and helps outperform in all life endeavors. However, good oral health is not just about owning this smile. Instead, it encompasses a mouth with strong teeth, healthy gums, a clean tongue, and good-smelling breath. According to the World Health Organization (WHO), oral health is a healthy state of mouth, orofacial structures, and teeth that supports an individual to perform all the necessary functions of life like eating, speaking, and breathing, which assists an individual to present themselves with great self-confidence and overall wellness along with the ability to socialize without the fears of embarrassment, discomfort, and pain (World Health Organization, 2023).

Moreover, good oral health provides immense positivity and willingness to an individual to engage in multifarious activities, interact with people, and enhance their potential beyond the limits. However, oral health doesn't remain the same throughout life and keeps changing based on different eating habits, lifestyle practices, health conditions, and hygiene levels. Oral health is not only a matter of concern for adults but also holds great significance in ensuring a healthy and happy life for young children, teenagers, and even older people. Thus, there is no defined age to care for and maintain good oral health that will eventually bless us with a healthy mouth and charming smile. On the whole, oral health is symbolic of one's overall personality and reflects the type of lifestyle one follows.

How is Oral Health Related to One's Overall Wellness?

In a health-oriented world, everyone is in the race to achieve good physical and mental health. As most of us choose the path of consuming a healthy diet and regular exercise, oral health is something that is left behind. Thus, being one of the neglected areas in the lives of most people, this makes it the biggest reason for the rising health issues, which eventually impact overall health. Based on the data provided by the World Health Organization for the year 2022, more than 3.5 billion individuals suffer from oral diseases globally, which is estimated to be three persons out of four (World Health Organization, 2022).

According to recent reports by the World Health Organization, around 2 billion people suffer from caries of permanent teeth, and 514 million kids suffer from caries of milk teeth worldwide (World Health Organization, 2022). Unfortunately, these oral health conditions are directly or indirectly linked to an individual's health. To our surprise, our mouth is the breeding place for numerous harmless bacteria, with about 700 species of oral bacteria living in our mouth alone, thereby contributing to an oral microbiome (Sahi, 2020). As long as these bacteria reside in the mouth area, they do not harm one's health. But, as the mouth is the entry point to the respiratory tract and digestive system of the body, it can become the number one cause of giving birth to diseases.

Brushing teeth regularly, flossing, and the body's natural defense system are the prime protectors that stop the bacteria from intervening with the smooth working of inner systems. However, poor hygiene habits can attract oral infections like gum diseases and tooth decay. Moreover, taking medicines like antidepressants, decongestants, diuretics, antihistamines, and painkillers reduces the flow of saliva, which eventually fails to neutralize the acids produced by the bacteria in the mouth and thus impacts overall health, thereby causing diseases. Thus, oral health is one of the most important factors contributing to maintaining good overall health and lifestyle.

Can Poor Oral Health Be Life-Threatening?

Oral health is one of the most neglected topics of concern for many individuals, as it is hard to believe they can ever get into an oral infection or problem. Poor oral hygiene can be linked to many diseases, while some may be serious and fatal. Sometimes, an oral disease called advanced periodontitis can impact the brain when associated with dementia and severe conditions such as Alzheimer's disease, resulting in memory loss. Oral infection can give rise to inflamed gums, which release substances harmful to killing the brain cells, resulting in memory problems. Further, gum diseases can also cause infertility in most women.

Gum issues can sometimes be serious, leading to complications for women who want to conceive or delay pregnancy. Gingivitis causes inflammation in the gums, which can spread inflammation to other parts of the body as well, triggering rheumatoid arthritis. In extreme cases, periodontal disease of the gums causes bacteria to enter the bloodstream, which leads to plaque building and hardening of the arteries, called atherosclerosis. This heart condition reduces the blood flow due to heart blockage, increasing the risk of heart attacks. Atherosclerosis damages blood vessels and arteries, which may result in hypertension, thus increasing the chances of strokes. This heart condition can sometimes lead to endocarditis, which happens when the infection reaches the lining of the heart and is a fatal condition.

It is very common for people with gum infections like periodontal disease to catch infection as they have weaker immune system function. Poor immunity is the root cause of serious kidney disease, which may be life-threatening due to the increased risk of kidney failure. Apart from this, poor oral hygiene also leads to the accumulation of oral bacteria, which increases the chances of premature death due to cancer. Ironically, sometimes, the simplest and easiest-looking things like oral health and hygiene could bring the worst harm to health. Thus, neglecting oral hygiene can cost your life, too.

Who Are Mostly Affected by Oral Health Issues?

Oral diseases are one of the common health issues that persist worldwide, affecting more than 45% of the world's population. The biggest challenge that causes such a high number of oral health issues is the lack of awareness. At the same time, socially disadvantaged and poor members of society are at higher risk of catching oral infections. Gum diseases are prevalent in people of all age groups and usually start from simple cavities, sensitivities, and pain that often turn into serious oral problems. Apart from this, people with poor oral hygiene, alcohol and tobacco use, and over-sugar consumption are at a higher risk of gum diseases.

How Often Should One Visit a Dentist?

No doubt, visiting a dentist sounds intimidating as it arouses the insecurity of different fears and pains within the mind. However, routine dental checkups are way too different than dental treatment, as the former is just an examination of oral health, while the latter is a specialized procedure for removing teeth, filling gaps, deep cleaning, and many more such issues. Thus, going for routine dental checkups is an easy and efficient way to prevent dental treatments. Dental checkups are a must for every individual, irrespective of their age and oral health condition. Regular visits to dentists help in finding out any oral health problems that may become severe and painful on negligence.

One of the biggest myths that keeps one from going to the dentist is that each sitting is painful. However, on a routine checkup, a dentist only performs a thorough examination of oral health and hygiene, followed by questions on eating habits, addictions, and advice and recommendations on good hygiene methods and treatment if required. There is no specific time to visit a dentist, but if you have healthy gums and teeth, it is good practice to visit at least twice a year. But, scheduling a dental checkup depends on many key factors like lifestyle and eating habits, hygiene attitude, family history and biological reasons, and accessibility to oral care products and services.

What Are the Must-Haves for a Healthy Mouth?

Achieving healthy gums and strong teeth is not an overnight process that can happen in a single go. Rather, accomplishing the goal of a healthy mouth needs consistent effort made with the right tips and tricks, along with regular dental checkups to ensure healthy gums and teeth. However, all this cannot happen on its own; instead, it requires a set of essential products that can help keep the cavities away and help in reaching optimal oral health. So, let's explore the list of oral health care must-haves to understand their significance and know the best way to use them for improving and maintaining good oral hygiene.

Probiotics

The mouth is home to large varieties of microbes, including several bacteria, some of which are beneficial, while the rest are harmful. Naturally, these microbes are present in a ratio that helps the good bacteria fight the bad ones. But sometimes, due to unfavorable conditions, the harmful bacteria multiply in number, which may begin to deteriorate the gum and teeth health, causing infections and diseases. In such circumstances, the supplements called probiotics can support eliminating harmful bacteria and promoting the functioning of good ones, thus supporting good oral health. Probiotics are healthy bacteria mostly used for improving gut health, but according to new research, they also support attaining a healthy oral cavity.

Probiotics can serve many benefits to oral health as they prevent plaque building, fight against bad breath, lower inflammation due to gum diseases, reduce the risk of oral cancers, and manage the symptoms of gum diseases like gingivitis. Probiotics are available in the form of natural food sources like soft cheese, milk, yogurt, and sour pickles. It is also found in the form of concentrated supplements like powder, pills, and mouthwash. It is recommended to take probiotics with prebiotics, which are substances high in fiber, and support these supplements to flourish in the intestines. Some of the prebiotics include raw honey, raw garlic, onion, and many more. Probiotics are usually safe for everyone but must be taken only on a doctor's recommendation. Furthermore, pregnant women, children, and seniors must avoid taking high levels of these supplements without the dentist's advice.

Toothbrush

Undoubtedly, the first thing that comes into one's mind while reflecting on oral hygiene is a toothbrush. But before selecting a toothbrush, it is necessary to explore and know the different types available in the market. The traditional manual toothbrush that has been in use for ages is one of the best ways to clean teeth, as it has a sturdy handle with flexible plastic bristles that come in varied stiffnesses like soft, medium, and hard.

However, in today's technology-oriented world, when one has the option of using smart electric brushes, this manual brush may seem to be a bit boring. Electric brushes are available in two different styles. Rotary electric brushes have a round head and remove plaque by their rotatory motion inside the mouth, whereas sonic electric brushes have an oval head that does the cleaning by its vibratory motion. Comparatively, a sonic electric brush is preferred for its better performance and coverage while cleaning the teeth. These brushes are available in different sizes for adults and kids.

Apart from this, one must be mindful while selecting a toothbrush, as using soft bristles helps prevent gum irritation, bleeding, and inflammation. For good oral hygiene, it is important to choose an anti-microbial self-cleaning toothbrush, which saves one from the hassles of keeping the toothbrush clean and free of bacteria. Moreover, one must check that the bristles of the toothbrush are thin so they can easily enter between the gumlines and teeth to get rid of any accumulated plaque or hardened bacteria.

Toothpaste

Just like a toothbrush is an essential need for maintaining good oral hygiene, choosing an appropriate toothpaste is also primary for healthy gums, preventing cavities and tooth decay. Brushing teeth without good toothpaste is not a good idea, as it does not scrub away the stubborn plaque and food particles from the teeth, thus triggering cavities and tooth problems. There are many different types of toothpaste available in the market based on the requirements of the user, like herbal toothpaste, traditional fluoride toothpaste, non-fluoride toothpaste, sensitivity toothpaste, and teeth whitening toothpaste.

Herbal toothpaste is free from artificial flavors and chemicals and is mainly made of natural ingredients derived from minerals and plants. Such a type of herbal toothpaste is suitable for individuals who are allergic to various chemicals found in other non-herbal toothpaste. Moreover, these herbal toothpastes are environment-friendly and not only provide protection from bacteria and mouth odor but also taste great. Despite the fact that herbal toothpaste is considered to be the best and healthful choice for both kids and adults, nowadays, other fluoride kinds of toothpaste are widely used for their instant results.

Apart from that, rising issues of cavities and tooth damage have increased the demand for sensitive toothpaste, which gives immediate relief from stinging tooth pain due to special ingredients like strontium chloride and potassium nitrate. Furthermore, the urge to own a beautiful and bright smile has compelled the crowd to try various teeth-whitening toothpaste, which shows appreciable results when used regularly in the long run.

Dental Floss

Using a toothbrush alone to clean the teeth on all sides is not enough to maintain healthy gums and mouth. Dental floss is an essential requirement that helps remove the small particles or debris stuck between the teeth. To maintain the best hygiene, floss your teeth regularly every night before brushing your teeth, as it helps in getting rid of any unwanted substances accumulated between the teeth and the gums. Dental floss is especially meant for people who struggle with cavities, have sensitive teeth, or have any allergies. Flossing after every meal helps in getting away with any food particles that may cause more problems and pain later.

Moreover, flossing can be done in varied ways, like using waxed and unwaxed flossers, the most common method to remove the debris stuck between the teeth. Super floss is beneficial for individuals with dental braces and wide gaps between the teeth and bridges. Floss picks can be the best option for people who are traveling as it is designed for single use only, which ensures hygiene and easy use. Apart from this, air flossers are also available, which use air pressure to push and remove the dirt and particles from between the teeth. Similarly, water flossers are also a great choice to eliminate unwanted food particles with the help of water pressure.

Toothpicks

Toothpicks, also called dental picks, are common in every home. The small, sleek pieces of wooden or plastic sticks are used for removing any hard bacteria, plaque, or food substance stuck in between the teeth and gums. These are of great help for the teeth at the sides where dental flossing fails to reach and provide effective results without any risk of allergies or pain. However, one must be careful while using the dental picks as the plastic or wooden stick would break off, causing injury if used with great pressure. This could be dangerous if it gets stuck firmly between the teeth, which must not be neglected as it could cause infection and pain.

Tongue Cleaner

In the whole process of caring for the teeth and gums, we often forget that taking care of the tongue is also a part of oral hygiene. Many of us don't know the main reason behind the foul or unpleasant smell that comes from the mouth. As a matter of fact, the bacteria that pile up on the tongue are majorly responsible for causing bad breath, which not only impacts health but also affects one's self-confidence and the ability to socialize in a negative manner. The most commonly used tool for cleaning the tongue effectively is the back part of the toothbrush, which has a rough surface for scrubbing away the dirt from the tongue easily. Moreover, a tongue scraper can also be used to remove any sort of debris from the tongue that not only freshens oral breath but also improves the functioning of taste buds by removing harmful germs and bacteria. Thus, it is considered a healthy habit to scrape the tongue at least once a day, along with brushing and flossing the teeth, in order to eliminate any bacteria build-up inside the mouth that can possibly cause gum inflammation, bad breath, and cavities.

Mouth Wash

Bad breath is one of the major issues faced by many people, which happens due to the bacteria present in the mouth that stays even after brushing teeth. Using mouthwash can help in solving the problem of bad breath easily. Regarding mouthwash, there are two types available in the market, one with alcohol and the other without alcohol. The non-alcoholic mouthwash is generally made up of natural mouth-freshening agents like mint, spearmint, peppermint, etc., which are mostly preferred as the alcoholic one results in drying of the gum tissues in the mouth and irritation, as well. Moreover, it is recommended to use mouthwash every time you brush your teeth, which removes the harmful bacteria that are left behind even after brushing. Furthermore, mouthwash is also available in many other varieties based on its purpose, like fluoride-based, antiseptic, and dry mouth.

Mouth Spray

Mouth freshener sprays are an important part of maintaining oral hygiene as they help kill the bacteria that toothbrushes and dental flossing cannot reach.

Mouth sprays also reduce bad breath in the mouth for approximately four hours. Mouth freshener sprays are available in many natural flavors based on their core ingredients, like cardamom, cinnamon, peppermint, spearmint, and many more.

Chapter 2:

Life-Changing Benefits of

Oral Health

Your smile is your logo; your personality is your business card.
Dental health is the foundation of your business. —Jay Danzie

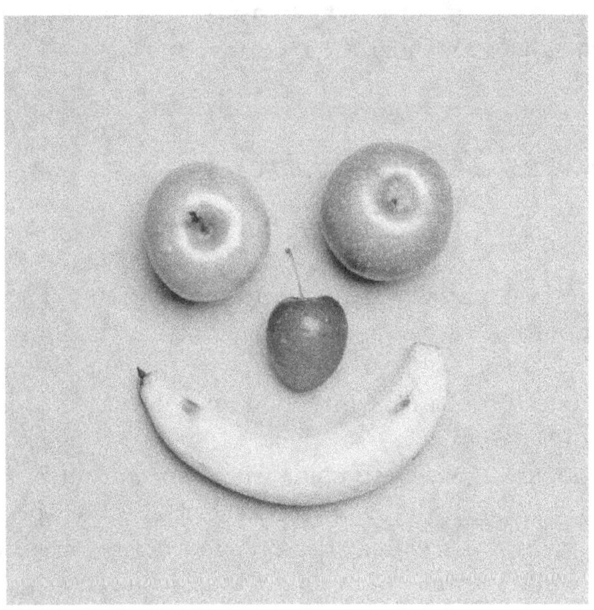

Since time immemorial, people have been keen enough
to improve their oral health for various reasons,

---

including beautifying themselves, maintaining hygiene, eliminating painful and unwanted symptoms of poor health, and many more. The need for maintaining good oral health is not only limited to the above-mentioned factors, as it can impact the life of a person in miraculous ways that are far beyond one's imagination and expectations. However, sometimes, mouth health is neglected, which may leave mild, severe, or irreversible impacts on the oral cavity and also the overall health. Knowing the various benefits and the key role that a good mouth plays in one's overall lifestyle can help inspire each individual to put in impactful and consistent effort to maintain and improve oral health. So, let's begin the journey to unveil the various ways in which a good mouth cavity transforms overall health by its life-changing benefits.

Retains Teeth Lifelong

Oral health and aging don't share an amazing relationship. As we age, we may encounter numerous health issues, some of which can be preventable while others can find a cure. Entering into old age, it is quite possible to avoid issues like arthritis, fatigue, and memory loss, while refraining from dental problems can be a challenging task. Teeth have resilient properties that help bear friction, pressure, and normal wear and tear while chewing and eating food. However, at times, the wear and tear are beyond the normal, which gradually degrades the quality of teeth while also affecting the inside of the mouth, corresponding to overall oral health. Apart from this, factors like poor hygiene and reluctance to follow and gain awareness about the importance of oral hygiene can cause irreversible loss of oral health.

All this eventually results in gum infections, teeth illness, periodontal disease, or tooth loss with aging, which makes it a compulsion for them to limit food choices, face speech issues, bear facial transformation, live poor social life due to isolation, and end up with degraded overall mental and physical health. However, practicing oral care from the very initial days can help reduce the risk of tooth loss and other oral infections and diseases with aging. The basics of oral hygiene, like brushing teeth twice a day, flossing, going for a routine dental checkup, and monitoring any negative signs or complications in dental health, could save one from the hassles of losing their teeth and getting into oral health problems as they grow old.

The best way to inculcate healthy oral hygiene habits is by practicing self-care, which compels one to be conscious about their everyday activities and lifestyle choices, which unknowingly and gradually impact their oral health without causing a sudden impact. Further, it is also important to gain knowledge about the significance and tips to maintain oral health, cut off negative addictive habits, and follow a balanced diet to get the appropriate nutrition that can boost oral health by strengthening the teeth. Giving up on addictions and improving habits can be a demanding task, but the inner drive to achieve good oral health can instill the motivation to bring the desired change to keep your teeth healthy for a lifetime.

Minimizes the Risk of Chronic Illness

Poor oral health and different types of chronic illness go hand in hand, as individuals suffering from oral issues are prone to chronic health diseases and vice versa. Research reveals that chronic diseases are the top underlying factors that cause disabilities and deaths in the United States (Mark, 2016). Common chronic issues like diabetes, health diseases, arthritis, obesity, and heart stroke are all linked with aggravating oral health problems. For instance, diabetes has remained an issue of puzzle for years, as it is difficult to decide which came first.

No doubt, diabetic people are easily susceptible to teeth loss and cavities, but in some cases, poor oral health is known for triggering chronic issues like diabetes. Often, infections are blamed for raising the blood sugar level. Likewise, gum infection can also increase the chances of developing diabetes. Similarly, gum diseases in the mouth are known for increasing inflammation, which is linked with a greater risk of cardiovascular problems like clogged arteries, heart strokes, and other heart diseases. Improving oral health is one of the effective ways to reduce the chances of developing any type of severe chronic illness.

Good oral health requires simple efforts but consistent efforts, most of which are related to avoiding unhealthy eating habits. For instance, quitting food that is high in sugar and fats helps lower the risk of diabetes. Apart from this, managing simple gum infections through regular dental checkups to reduce inflammation can also reduce the risk of getting caught in unwanted cardiovascular diseases. Restricting intake of alcohol and tobacco and improving diet is the key to achieving healthy gums and mouth, which automatically cuts down the dangers of chronic diseases.

Boosts Self-Confidence

Self-confidence is the ability of a person to believe in their skills, potential, and worth that makes them stand out in the crowd and helps them accomplish goals. It is that single vital quality that can save you from failures as it fills in the required courage to strive repeatedly until you win. Self-confidence is that inner voice that helps a person to move closer to better opportunities and individuals without any fear or hesitation. However, poor self-confidence can directly impact an individual's mental state and make them feel unworthy of trying new and better things, restricting their ability to explore the hidden potential.

Self-confidence is directly related to the way a person perceives themselves, while good oral health plays a critical role in this. Oral health issues like crooked teeth, yellowish teeth, or tooth loss can impact how a person looks at oneself, drastically reducing their inner confidence and making them feel bad about themselves. Apart from this, the pain and discomfort caused by dental problems can cause dissatisfaction, directly impacting their participation in personal, professional, and social life. However, adopting healthy oral hygiene habits, routine dental checkups, and other precautionary measures to improve oral health can boost self-confidence, making one feel stress-free, happier, and optimistic about themselves and the situation.

Good oral health opens the gate to a fearless journey where there is no place for anxiety and negative thoughts that stop them from achieving targets. Self-confidence is the most important ingredient to a successful life, filling in the required motivation to pursue dreams and make them happen. Therefore, putting in the right and consistent efforts to keep one's teeth free of germs and bacteria, getting rid of bad breath, discoloration or yellowing of teeth, and other mouth-related issues can help in making them feel confident from within that never fails to reflect on the outside, making all the difference.

Gives a Beautiful Smile

Achieving a beautiful white smile that marks perfection is the dream and expectation of every individual. A sparkling white smile is often the set beauty standard that marks the definition of flawlessness and symbolizes healthy oral health. However, a shining smile does not necessarily mean being a faultless one, as these white-looking teeth are vulnerable to gum diseases and cavities, just like the ones that are not as bright and perfect.

Beauty has often been misinterpreted with neat and clean, pearly white smiles that look the most attractive to catch the attention of the crowd. However, a good smile is the one that forms an epitome of health as well as beauty, which not only has outer looks and perception of perfection but is beautiful inside out. Efforts to maintain and improve oral health are one of the effective ways to achieve a healthy and beautiful smile that can make you stand out. When talking about a beautiful smile, one must not be confined to achieving healthy, white, and strong teeth. Moreover, it also includes the gums free of pain and any sort of infections and diseases.

Confidence is a major role player that adds moon and stars to one's smile, making them look more beautiful. However, bad breath and crooked teeth are the barriers that can steal away confidence and fill in the unwanted doubt and consciousness in a person, impacting the way they carry and portray themselves. A beautiful smile is the secret to conquering the world because it makes you believe in your capabilities by reducing stress and self-doubt while enhancing mood and mental health and making one more successful on personal and professional fronts.

Enhances Personality

Personality is the representation of external traits and qualities of an individual that differentiates them from others. Personality is the first thing that comes into notice when you enter a crowded room. It is that vital characteristic that can make a person stand out among the crowd, eventually making them feel more special, empowered, confident, and worthy. People with good personalities are known for creating strong relationships wherever they go, be it their personal life or professional.

Personality is a feature that makes a person look more attractive and makes them feel wanted, which drives their self-esteem to the best level. However, the first thing that could impact one's personality is their appearance. Oral health plays a significant role in determining the personality of an individual as it is the most prominent thing to be noticed by one and all. A person with broken or yellowish teeth, foul breath, or any kind of visible gum disease or cavities would never be able to feel comfortable, which automatically degrades their personality and looks. Personality is how you carry yourself and can be surely built and enhanced with time. However, poor oral health and severe oral illness could make it a demanding task for one to groom oneself and improve their outer personality. Individuals who are conscious about themselves and their looks and have a deep desire to outperform others have a special focus on their overall health, which includes personality development too.

Maintaining and improving oral health and hygiene is the foremost step to building a better, pleasing, and charming personality that doesn't fail to impress others at a single sight. Therefore, oral health not only provides inner motivation, self-confidence, and a beautiful smile but also makes you look presentable and unique, distinctively, and specially.

Provides Overall Wellness

In the race of life, every mortal is striving hard to achieve good health by improving their lifestyle and adopting the best habits. However, most of the time, oral health remains ignored, as it is hard for one to relate between oral health and overall wellness. Good health is not just about a proper physical body that can be achieved by regular exercise, balanced food, and giving up on addictions.

Overall, health is all about having a stress-free life without psychological pressure or illness, making one feel at their best. However, oral health is part of our overall fitness that is often neglected, which not only deteriorates and degrades physical health but also causes mental health problems, eventually affecting their ability to form strong bonds with people around them. A mind free of stress and negative self-perception can achieve good mental and physical wellness, positively impacting their social well-being.

Poor oral health is the root cause of creating an imbalance in all the important aspects of life, viz., physical, mental, and social well-being. However, a little investment into good oral hygiene practices can help one achieve an enhanced physical body with reduced risk of chronic illness like diabetes, cardiovascular disease, obesity, and cancer. Further, better oral health is directly related to a positive state of mind as it makes one feel good about themselves, raising self-esteem. People with good oral and physical health have a relaxed state of mind, which is the foremost requirement for developing strong and cordial relations with people in their personal and professional lives. Therefore, directly, or indirectly, oral health has a big role to play in the overall wellness of an individual.

Reduces Dental Visits

It is always intimidating for one to visit a dentist, mostly due to the misconception that regular visits can be painful, causing anxiety and fear. However, routine dental visits can be much more beneficial and less painful as they help save you from the trauma, agony, and discomfort of dental treatments. Dental treatments are unavoidable situations that are created due to negligence and poor oral hygiene practices, ending up in severe and complicated oral health problems.

Many oral health issues like cavities, gum inflammation, gum bleeding, dental caries, tooth loss, and periodontal disease need urgent treatment, which compels one to rush to a dentist to soothe and relieve the pain. Treatments like getting rid of a cavity or extracting a tooth due to severe infection are extremely painful, which adds to a torturous dental experience. However, being mindful from the beginning and putting in consistent efforts to improve one's oral health can help in reducing dental visits and treatments. Some oral self-care methods like brushing teeth twice daily, flossing every night, using mouthwash and spray, limiting addictive habits of tobacco and smoking, and many more are simple ways to boost oral health.

Apart from this, consulting a dentist for oral health scanning at least twice a year is an effective and practical way to ensure good oral health. Routine dental checkups have many benefits, such as helping in the early detection of problems, saving from the discomfort of treatment and tooth extraction, resolving bad breath issues, and making one feel more confident, satisfied, and assured about their good oral health.

Saves Pennies

Oral health issues are not only scary and painful but could also cost you much. Good oral health holds a strong relationship with dental costs, and the more you invest in dental care and hygiene practices, the more money you save. It is obvious that a healthy mouth helps you to escape discomfort as well as save an extra penny. Thus, it is important to understand the deep-rooted connection between these factors. Routine preventive dental care and visits can help reduce treatment costs by up to ten times. Following the key steps for improving oral health automatically reduces the need to treat future dental problems.

Apart from this, dental treatments and high costs are not limited to the initial treatment. Instead, some of the dental restorations like dentures, crown replacement, and filling need timely replacement, adding to more cost. Further, poor oral health also aggravates many physical and mental health conditions like stress and anxiety, heart health issues, diabetes, and many more. However, with proper care and early preventive measures, one can easily avoid getting into situations that require high-cost and periodic treatment.

Chapter 3:

Red Flags of Poor Oral Hygiene

A genuine smile comes from the heart, but a healthy smile needs good dental care. - Wayne Chirisa

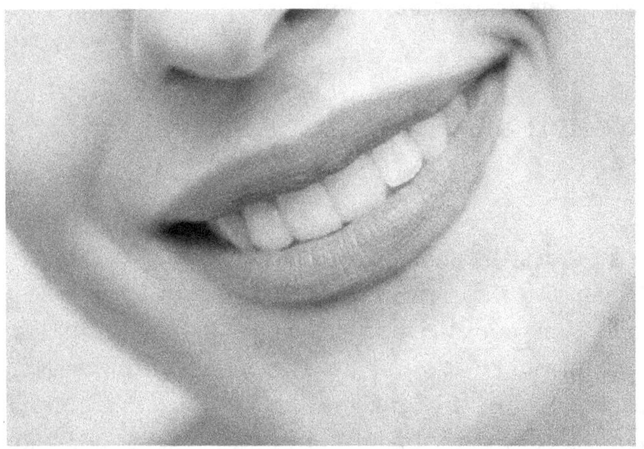

Developing good health is gaining importance in a world full of beauty and wellness freak people. The fundamental to attaining this goal requires following a healthy lifestyle with good eating habits, apt nutrition, regular exercise, sleep hygiene, and many more. However, the journey to a healthy lifestyle is incomplete without the right investment in maintaining good oral health. Developing a healthy mouth and a sane body are directly or indirectly linked with each other, as one cannot achieve overall wellness without a healthy mouth and vice versa. But sometimes, this endeavor is full of obstacles, including a lack of awareness. Having no idea about the simple signs and symptoms of the impacted oral health leads to negligence in seeking preventive measures, which results in the deterioration of gums and teeth, gradually affecting the whole body. However, with prior knowledge about the red flags of poor oral health, it becomes easy to opt for the right preventive actions and treatment. So, let's delve into and discover the various red flags that indicate poor oral health that will make it easier to achieve a perfect smile.

Swollen and Bleeding Gums

In the quest to achieve a healthy mouth, the attention of many of us is driven toward strong and pearly teeth, while gums are the most neglected part. Healthy gums are important for good oral health and impact overall health. Most of the time, swollen and bleeding gums are the greatest indication of gum illness. Thus, consulting a dentist is the best way to determine the main causes of sore and painful gums. In some cases, swollen and bleeding gums are not due to any disease but due to negligent oral hygiene habits. One of the most common causes of painful and bleeding gums is the wrong way of brushing teeth. Always choose a toothbrush with soft bristles, and brush teeth in a circular motion.

Using hard or medium bristles and brushing harshly back and forth can damage the enamel on the tooth, resulting in soreness and swollen gums. Apart from this, incorrect flossing techniques can also hurt your gums, which may cause them to bleed, swell, and pain. Further, severe gum diseases like gingivitis and periodontitis are also the underlying cause of swollen and bleeding gums. Research reveals that more than 47% of Americans aged 30 or older suffer from some gum illness called periodontal disease (Parker, 2022). Canker sores are mouth ulcers that can happen anywhere in the mouth and are responsible for causing discomfort to the gums, causing gum bleeding, and swelling.

Pain in Teeth and Gums

Teeth pain is common among children, adults, and older people, which is an indication of any problem with their oral health. Teeth ache does not necessarily mean that it is a severe problem because, at times, minor oral issues can also cause much pain. Teeth ache feels like a sharp tingling sensation at irregular intervals or can be persistent throughout the time. Pain in teeth can cause extreme discomfort, disrupt your peace of mind and sleep, cause stress, and make you feel uneasy throughout the day. At times, when tooth pain persists for a longer period, it becomes a necessity to visit a dentist to enquire about the oral health problem.

Many reasons cause pain in teeth and gums, including gum diseases, sensitivity in teeth, decaying of teeth, impacted teeth, cracked teeth, and pulpitis, also called tooth pulp inflammation. Teeth pain must never be neglected at the initial stages as the precautionary and preventive measures are efficient enough to heal the issues, while prolonged pain in gum and teeth can result in serious oral issues, which may take time to get better.

Loose Teeth

As a kid, experiencing loose teeth is quite common and is less concerning because it is a normal process for replacing milk teeth with permanent ones. However, loose teeth can be concerning for adults as it is a sign that the teeth are losing support from the gums and bone, which may slowly be detached permanently. Loose teeth in adults are followed by many other complications like red and swollen gums, bleeding gums, and gums recession. At times, loose teeth happen due to an injury, while in other cases, it is an indication of any severe oral disease. The first sign of loss of teeth is visible during brushing teeth when you feel like they are wobbling and causing pain.

It mostly happens when any type of bacterial infection becomes severe and attacks your tissues, gums, and bones surrounding the teeth. Poor oral hygiene is the major cause of gum disease, which starts from degrading gum health, making them red, swollen, and bleeding, eventually affecting the bone and deteriorating teeth health. Loose teeth can be reversed if one opts for early detection and treatment of the problem. Some of the common treatments for loose teeth based on the severity of gum disease are bone grafting, flap surgery, bite adjustment, splinting, and mouth guard.

Tooth Sensitivity

Teeth sensitivity is a common sign of oral health problems that many individuals experience. It is not strange to feel a sharp tingling sensation each time you eat something cold or hot food. Tooth sensitivity, also called dentin hypersensitivity, makes one feel extreme discomfort and pain in response to outside stimuli, often cold and hot temperatures. Teeth sensitivity may affect one tooth, many, or all teeth depending on the hygiene and oral care routine. However, in the initial stages, teeth sensitivity can be easily treated by adopting healthy oral care measures recommended by the dentist.

Sensitivity can be triggered due to cold air, hot or cold food, sweet food, acidic food, alcohol-based mouthwash, cold water, or while flossing and brushing teeth. The major cause of sensitivity is the thinning down of the enamel that protects the teeth, while some people who naturally have thin enamel can have more sensitive teeth. However, common causes of wearing enamel are grinding teeth, using a hard bristle toothbrush, brushing with force, and regularly consuming acidic food and drinks.

Plaque Formation

Plaque is a sticky, thin coating that is formed on the teeth every day. This coating feels slippery and fuzzy on the surface of your teeth each morning when you get up. Research has found that plaque is a layer of living microbes, and a gluey textured polymer layer often surrounds this community. This sticky layer is the means that helps the microbes to attach to the teeth surface, which multiplies into microcolonies. Plaque formation is unhealthy for the teeth as it provides a healthy environment for the bacteria to grow and thrive in. These piled-up bacteria produce acids that are harmful to the teeth and result in tooth decay.

Negligence and poor hygiene lead to the accumulation of plaque, which can cause the minerals from saliva to form a hard yellow layer called tartar. Prolonged plaque formation leads to tartar building at the gumline, both at the back and front teeth. Initially, plaque is transparent and cannot be seen by the naked eye, while it is a breeding place for bacteria causing infections and oral diseases. Regular flossing and brushing teeth are simple and effective ways to get rid of initial plaque formed in the teeth, while to get rid of hard plaque and tartar, it is important to have a dental cleaning with a dental hygienist or dentist.

Dry Mouth

Dry mouth, as the name suggests, is an oral health condition in which the salivary glands in the mouth fail to produce enough saliva that is necessary to keep it healthy. This condition, also called xerostomia, causes a dry feeling in the mouth that may result in other oral issues like bad breath, cracked lips, and dry throat. Saliva is very important for the proper digestion of food as it supports moistening and breaking down the food we eat. Saliva also ensures that the gums and teeth are in good health while combating the risk of any tooth decay, mouth sores, or gum diseases.

Usually, dry mouth is not an alarming oral problem, but it may be a sign of any other severe health issues that must be considered. Dry mouth may be caused by many factors like poor hydration, radiation therapy, side effects of any medication, too much anxiety and stress, snoring and mouth breathing, aging, or smoking tobacco. Apart from this, many other medical conditions are also responsible for causing dry mouth, like diabetes, Alzheimer's disease, nerve damage, or oral thrush. Oral thrush is a type of yeast infection inside the mouth, which leads to inflammation and damaging the salivary glands, disabling these glands to produce enough saliva.

Bad Breath

Bad breath is an oral health condition that causes a foul smell in the mouth, while in some cases, it may also cause a bad taste. In some situations, the bad taste in the mouth is due to the food we eat, which usually goes away after brushing our teeth or using mouthwash. But the bad taste caused by the bad breath condition may not disappear even after struggles with mouthwash and rinsing. General causes of bad breath are poor oral hygiene, consuming food and beverages with a strong odor, having a dry mouth, smoking, periodontal disease, plaque formation, throat or mouth condition, and sinus.

Sometimes, bad breath is also caused due to some underlying diseases like diabetes, kidney issues, liver diseases, or gastric disorders. Making small dental hygiene changes can help eliminate bad breath, for instance, brushing twice daily, flossing after each meal, and drinking lots of water. However, if bad breath persists even after efforts of improved oral hygiene habits, then it is time to see a doctor because there can be any severe health condition causing bad odor.

Mouth Ulcers

Mouth sores, also called canker sores, are small painful lesions that occur inside the mouth or at the base of the gums due to sensitivities, allergies, or injuries. Mouth ulcers do not spread and usually go away on their own, but these may cause extreme discomfort and pain while eating, drinking, or talking. Accidental bites, injury from hard brushing or dental work, or dental braces can cause mouth ulcers. Sometimes, bacteria, oral infections, or allergies can also cause painful mouth sores. Hormonal changes, emotional stress, improper sleep, or deficiency of vitamin B12, B9, iron, and folate can also develop mouth ulcers.

Apart from this, other health conditions like inflammatory bowel syndrome, celiac disease, and diabetes can also be responsible for causing mouth ulcers. Mouth sores can be prevented by avoiding acidic and spicy food, which can aggravate them, while including a balanced diet and multivitamin supplements helps in improving overall oral health. Use a toothbrush with soft bristles and brush teeth gently to prevent mouth sores due to accidental biting and injuries in the mouth. Following healthy sleep and oral hygiene habits along with reduced stress are the other helpful ways to avoid mouth ulcers.

Chapter 4

Risk Factors of Poor Oral Health

Good dental hygiene leads to overall well-being. — common phrase

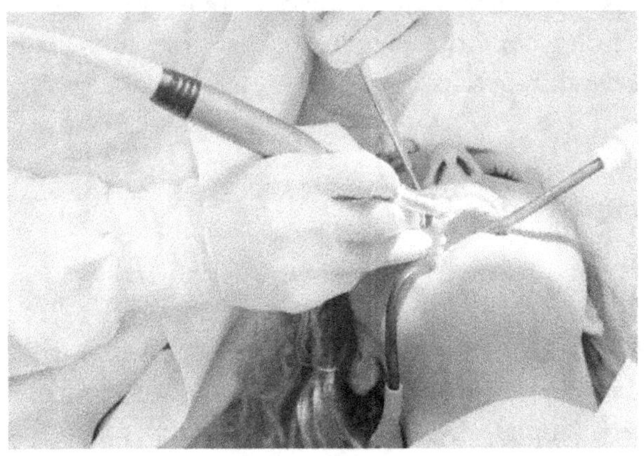

The oral cavity is the delicate and most important part of our body as it supports the key functions crucial in day-to-day life like intake of the apt nutrition, communication, breakdown of food, and ensuring overall wellness. Negligence to maintain good oral health, unhealthy addictive habits, and poor lifestyle can lead to many complications in the mouth that range from mild to severe. However, there are many other serious health issues that directly or indirectly impact the oral cavity and can trigger dental illness and complications.

Lack of awareness about the major health issues that can have adverse consequences in the oral cavity leads to irresponsible and negligent behavior toward maintaining a healthy mouth. With the knowledge of the risk factors that can aggravate oral health conditions, it becomes easier to seek the appropriate medical advice at the right time that can save one from getting serious mouth problems. So, let's start the endeavor to gain an in-depth idea about the various risk factors and their serious impacts that are linked with oral health conditions to create ease for one to combat their harsh repercussions.

Type-2 Diabetes

Our body is a closed system that works well unless any outside foreign particle in the form of viruses and bacteria enters the system and interrupts its smooth functioning. The only outer way for harmful bacteria to enter the body and circulatory system is through open wounds in the skin, lungs, and mouth. Most people fail to understand the importance of the mouth when it comes to catching infections and inviting chronic diseases. The mouth is home to a large number of bacteria, which may be harmful to human health as well. Negligence to take proper care of oral health and hygiene can create adverse conditions inside the body, as the bacteria find a way to breach the smooth functioning of the body through the bloodstream.

Oral health diseases like gingivitis, periodontal disease, and dental caries are critical mouth conditions that develop because of the multiplication of harmful bacteria due to poor oral care and hygiene. These dental problems can lead to bleeding gums, eroding of tooth enamel, and weakening of bones and teeth, which makes it easy for harmful bacteria to enter the circulatory system. Diabetes is a medical condition that can get worse due to oral bacterium. Research claims that inflammation caused in the mouth and gum due to dental diseases reduces the ability of the body to utilize the insulin in the blood and manage blood sugar (Jovinally, 2015).

This condition can aggravate the problem as it begins a cycle where oral bacteria increase blood sugar levels, while high blood sugar provides a perfect medium for bacteria to grow and thrive in. Further, poor oral health and diabetes share a strong relationship, as diabetes weakens immunity and increases the chances of getting trapped in gum infection and oral diseases, and vice versa. Thus, it is important to maintain good oral health to reduce the threat of diabetes, while people with diabetes must invest in extra oral care as they are at a greater risk of oral health diseases.

Heart Diseases

Oral health diseases are painful and cause physical discomfort in the mouth but can also cause severe problems in other body parts. According to the World Health Organization, cardiovascular disease is one of the major concerns as it is responsible for causing the maximum number of deaths annually, estimated at 17.9 million every year (World Health Organization, 2022a). Cardiovascular disease is linked to problems in blood vessels and the heart, which increases the risk of coronary heart disease, rheumatic heart disease, cerebrovascular diseases, and other severe conditions. At the same time, the maximum number of cardiovascular deaths is due to heart strokes and heart attacks.

The major causes of heart disease include an inactive lifestyle, an imbalanced diet, excessive use of tobacco and alcohol, and clogged or blocked arteries. Poor oral health is one of the major reasons that can cause blocked arteries or clogging in the bloodstream, a condition called atherosclerosis. Negligence about maintaining a healthy mouth can lead to the accumulation of bacteria in the mouth due to plaque formation. In some conditions, the bacteria in the plaque can cause inflammation of the gums, which affects the bloodstream and can lead to plaque building in the arteries.

Accumulating plaque in the arteries can harden them, blocking the bloodstream and raising blood pressure, eventually increasing the risk of heart attacks. However, this extreme situation can be controlled if instant dental treatment is taken. Following proper oral hygiene by brushing teeth and flossing daily, along with getting consistent dental treatment to eliminate harmful bacteria, can help prevent the adverse scenarios of heart attacks. Therefore, oral health must not be neglected, as simple problems of the mouth can turn into life-threatening medical conditions, which makes it difficult for one to strive through and prevent the consequences.

Respiratory Diseases

Oral health is important as it enhances the beauty and confidence within a person. However, it can be a challenging task to maintain oral health due to lack of knowledge, unavailability of resources, and unawareness about the complications it may cause. Oral health is not just limited to bright, shining teeth, but it is also associated with the overall wellness of individuals. Research proclaims that poor oral health is responsible for causing acute lung diseases like pneumonia and bronchitis. Negligence toward maintaining good oral hygiene can also aggravate an already existing respiratory disease.

According to research, poor oral health and respiratory diseases are strongly linked because sometimes lung disease can also cause the loss of tooth enamel, increased risk of oral illness, and negative impact on the teeth and gums, and vice versa. Oral health issues like gingivitis and tooth decay are caused by the germs and bacteria in the plaque formed on the teeth. During teeth infection, some harmful bacteria may travel down the respiratory tract and lungs, causing an infection. Plaque formed at the teeth is the breeding home of bacteria as its environment is friendly enough, which helps multiply them.

At times, these bacteria can be inhaled by the lungs in the form of tiny drops of saliva. In such situations, it is easy for healthy lungs to fight the infections caused by such bacteria. However, already infected lungs are not that strong and immune to the harsh effects of oral bacteria, complicating and increasing the risk factor of infections and worsening the condition. Gum infections are responsible for raising inflammation in the respiratory airways, which is the major cause of lung damage and shows severe symptoms. Thus, inflammation and infection in the gums often signal an alarming sign to the other parts of the body, including the lungs. However, appropriate action taken to combat gum diseases and inflammation can help improve the condition of the lungs and teeth.

Dementia or Alzheimer's Disease

Protecting teeth and gums is an integral part of flourishing your oral health and avoiding any kind of painful infections or diseases. Oral bacteria in the mouth not only impact your oral health but can also show adverse effects on the brain, resulting in memory loss. Apt functioning of brain cells is important not just to ensure the proper working of the other parts of the body but also because it is directly linked with memory; however, as a person ages, memory loss becomes a major issue faced by most individuals, which can have many causes.

Mostly, memory issues stem from the brain itself, but in some cases, poor oral hygiene can also become the triggering factor, which may lead to problems in remembering things. Memory is an important part of our overall working system as it helps to perform various key functions of life without any complications. But the loss of memory, especially with aging, can become a huge obstacle in the way to their participation in important activities. Research reveals that periodontal disease is very common in senior adults above the age of 65 years. This disease affects more than 70% of individuals over the age of 65 and is characterized by systemic and chronic inflammation within the pockets between the teeth and the gums, which is the breeding place of bacteria, increasing the chances of developing memory problems.

According to research, more than 85% of senior patients with memory loss issues have been diagnosed with oral issues and not Alzheimer's disease. The bacteria invading the oral space due to periodontal disease causes inflammation in the gums, which sometimes enter into the bloodstream and may also cause damage to the brain tissues, eventually impacting memory with aging. Overall, the ability to maintain oral hygiene declines, which may result in such adverse conditions. However, awareness, proper attention, and consistent effort can help avoid any type of oral disease and prevent such chronic illness in other parts of the body.

Oral Cancer

Oral health is often not considered a serious issue by most people due to a belief that poor oral hygiene has only adverse impacts in the form of gum and teeth infections, which can be treated. However, poor oral hygiene can sometimes turn into a dangerous health condition called cancer. Normal and healthy cells in the body have a lifecycle in which they grow, multiply, and die. However, when some cells in the oral cavity become abnormal, they don't follow the regular lifecycle and multiply rapidly, which eventually results in oral cancer. These abnormal cancer cells are strong enough to invade the healthy cells in the mouth, damaging the healthy tissue in this process. The oral cavity comprises lips, gums, teeth, the inside of the mouth, the base of the mouth, and the roof and bottom of the mouth. The primary and most sensitive spots of developing oral cancer are the lips, bottom of the tongue, and inside of the mouth.

According to research, poor oral hygiene and unhealthy eating habits causing adverse mouth health conditions are the biggest causes of developing oral cancers (Everett, 2022). Individuals who consume alcohol, tobacco, and smoke are at a greater risk of developing cancer, as it becomes difficult for them to maintain good oral hygiene. Research reveals that improving the oral cavity helps in reducing the risk of developing oral cancers (Everett, 2022). Going for regular dental visits, brushing teeth more than twice a day, and preventing tooth decay can help reduce the chances of poor oral health. Apart from this, consuming a balanced and nutritious diet and restricting the use of tobacco, alcohol, and other addictions can also minimize the risk of oral cancer. Opting for a regular oral cancer screening is also an important preventive measure for individuals addicted to alcohol and tobacco, as early detection of a problem can save them from harsh and irreversible impacts.

Periodontal Diseases

Periodontal disease is a common oral health problem that affects the gums and bones in the oral cavity. This disease causes inflammation and infection in the tissues that surround and hold the teeth firmly attached to the gums. Healthy teeth and gums don't cause pain and discomfort, but with periodontal disease, swelling, and bleeding, gums are a common issue that may result in discoloration of gums into purplish or reddish color. When periodontal disease is left untreated, it results in the destruction and weakening of the jawbone and tissue in that area, eventually leading to tooth loss. It is difficult to identify periodontal disease in the initial stages as the guns and teeth do not have swelling, pain, or bleeding. Therefore, having an in-depth knowledge about oral disease and its various stages can help in improving the situation by adopting the right prevention and treatment.

The first stage of periodontal disease often shows signs like puffy and painful gums that may bleed during flossing and brushing teeth. This stage is called gingivitis, a reversible oral condition by adopting apt care and treatment. In the second stage, called a mild stage, the bacteria sweep inside the gums, which impacts the supporting bones. During this stage, the gums are pulled away from the teeth, creating pockets that become breeding and hiding places for the bacteria and making it difficult to remove them through flossing and brushing. The third stage is moderate periodontal disease, which erodes the ligaments, soft tissues, and bones, holding the teeth firmly. This stage is marked by bad breath, pain, and pus around the gumline.

The last and advanced stage is marked with loss and painful tooth that also results in tooth loss in worse cases. The major reason that may cause periodontal disease is poor oral hygiene. Improper oral care leads to plaque accumulation on the teeth layer that provides a friendly environment for harmful oral bacteria to breed and multiply in number. Apart from this, some individuals' genes are responsible for reducing immunity, which makes it difficult for the self-defense of the oral cavity to prevent periodontal diseases even after efforts to maintain good oral health. Other risk factors like consuming tobacco, alcohol, smoking, stress, diabetes, autoimmune disease, and heart disease also increase the risk of periodontal disease.

Osteoporosis

Osteoporosis is a medical condition that occurs with aging and impacts bone density and strength, making them susceptible to fractures. This health condition is more common among women than in men and is also deeply associated with aging. As we age, the bones become less dense, making them weaker, which increases the risk of falling, bone breaking, stooped posture, back pain, and loss of height. The major risk factors of osteoporosis are hormonal changes, especially at the time of menopause among aging women. Medical conditions like rheumatoid arthritis also increase the chances of developing osteoporosis.

Apart from this, research has proclaimed that weak teeth and poor oral health are also strongly linked with causing osteoporosis. The risk factors of oral health and osteoporosis are common, including hormonal imbalance, poor nutrition, unhealthy diet, and aging. Gum disease, called periodontal disease, is a bacterial infection that directly impacts the teeth and the tissue surrounding them. The formation of the plaque helps these bacteria to thrive, which becomes adverse and can also result in tooth loss and jawbone loss. According to research, individuals with periodontal disease have lower bone density in the jaw bones, which is a sign of osteoporosis and eventually results in tooth loss.

Routine dental checkup helps in identifying the underlying issues of lost and painful teeth, which ensures prevention and apt treatment. A diet rich in vitamin D and calcium provides the appropriate nutrient that improves bone and teeth health. Apart from this, doing regular exercise, getting rid of addictions like tobacco, and following proper oral hygiene methods are simple ways to avoid and combat oral diseases that are linked with osteoporosis.

Obesity

Obesity is a serious health condition that increases body fat abnormally and is a matter of concern globally. Most of us believe that obesity is caused by unhealthy eating habits only. However, many other factors actively contribute to being overweight. Poor oral health is one such element that is linked with causing obesity in individuals. Poor oral hygiene increases the risk of gum infections and diseases, which reduces the ability to taste food and results in overeating, eventually causing overweight. Further, oral illnesses like periodontal disease make it difficult to consume a normal diet. Eating a restricted diet results in consuming food rich in calories but low in nutrients, thus causing weight gain.

Periodontal disease is also known for causing inflammation throughout the body, which leads to hormonal imbalance, thus increasing the appetite and lowering the energy levels. Apart from this, oral health disrupts the normal working of the digestive system, which restricts the ability of the body to absorb nutrients. Poor digestion often leads to malnutrition, which may cause obesity. Poor oral health is also an underlying cause of diabetes in most individuals, which makes it difficult for the body to control the blood sugar level, leading to extreme hunger and obesity. Therefore, investing in healthy oral hygiene habits, consuming a balanced and nutritious diet, and doing regular exercises can help reduce the risk of both oral diseases and obesity.

Chapter 5

Barriers on The Path of Achieving Oral Health

Good oral hygiene is a gift you give to yourself. —common phrase

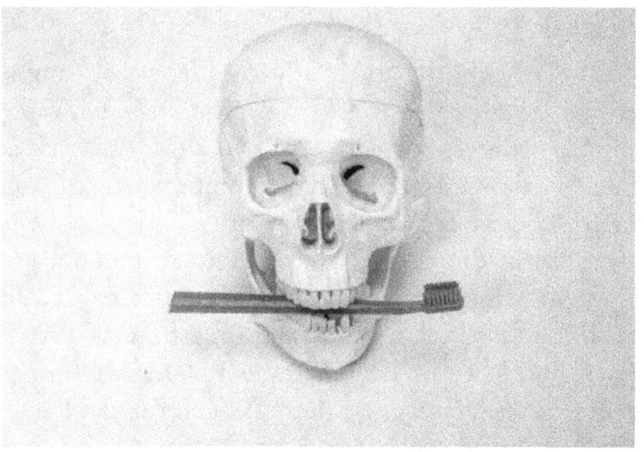

Attaining good oral health requires consistent efforts and a set of effective habits that make the entire process simple and easy to follow. However, sometimes, the journey of maintaining a healthy mouth can become a tricky one due to the various obstacles that may come in the way in the form of unhealthy eating habits, addictions, past traumatic experiences, and unavoidable diseases. Further, at times, factors like lack of information and inaccessibility to dental hygiene essentials make it difficult for one to put in the right efforts that are necessary for good oral health. However, having an idea about these barriers can open the gates that can help one avoid falling into the trap of negligent habits and unavoidable circumstances. So, let's explore, analyze, and understand the most common hurdles that one may encounter on the journey of achieving good oral and overall health.

Improper Eating Habits

Often, in the hurly and burly of life, to accomplish personal and professional responsibilities with great zeal, one fails to neglect one's health. Physical and mental health are the major components of one's overall wellness. However, most often forget to include oral health in the checklist. Failure to maintain a good oral cavity can also lead to health problems in other parts of the body. Diet is an important factor that can impact not just physical and mental health but also dental wellness. However, the food you eat can become the biggest hurdle on the path to achieving good dental health.

Unhealthy eating habits like consuming sugary drinks, acidic and sweetened foods and drinks, and non-nutritious snacks create an unfavorable environment in the oral cavity. Improper diet has direct, harsh impacts on the teeth and oral cavity, causing tooth decay, bad breath, and other severe diseases like periodontitis and oral cancers. Apart from this, improper eating habits also impact the inner tissues. Lack of the appropriate nutrients makes it quite challenging for the inner tissues to bear the infection, and they become more prone to gum diseases and tooth decay. Transforming and adopting healthy eating habits can alone make a great difference in oral health, creating ease for one to achieve healthy gums and teeth.

Lack of Awareness

In the haze to achieve a beautiful smile, we often fail to overlook the essentials that form the base of good oral health. One of the crucial factors that most of us fail to excel in is basic dental knowledge and awareness, which is a must for maintaining overall health. Having less or no knowledge about dental hygiene habits makes it difficult for most individuals to practice the right steps to maintain their oral health. Lack of awareness leads to poor and ineffective oral hygiene efforts, the prime reason for bad breath, plaque building, cavities, and many other problems. Without knowing the perks of flossing, using mouthwash, regular dental visits, and the right way of brushing teeth, oral hygiene efforts and the health impacts remain an unrealized and ignored problem among people.

Many oral health issues show their first signs and symptoms in the form of mild dental issues like slight gum pain, bleeding, and sensitivity. Still, a lack of awareness can cause negligence to reflect on those problems and are left untreated for time, which may turn into severe medical conditions. Apart from this, visiting the dentist is perceived to be a treatment need rather than a preventive dental behavior, which transforms mild oral health symptoms into gum infections and diseases. Therefore, general awareness about dental health, initial signs and symptoms, preventive measures, and the importance of routine dental visits are key to building a healthy mouth and sane body.

Financial Crisis

Achieving a healthy mouth is an easy task with apt knowledge about the importance and varied ways of maintaining oral health. But sometimes, there are unavoidable barriers in life that can create much difficulty for one to put in efforts to maintain good oral health. Financial crisis is one such obstacle that comes in the way of developing a healthy oral cavity. Financial crisis not only makes it challenging to obtain the best resources to clean, floss, brush, and maintain a healthy mouth, but it also creates difficulty in getting timely dental health care. According to research, more than half of Americans delay their dental and other medical care due to financial problems (University of Illinois Chicago, 2019). Further, around 80% of Americans delay their dental treatment and care procedures due to the higher costs it would levy in the future.

Poor oral hygiene due to the inability to afford basic dental essentials like good quality toothbrushes, apt toothpaste, floss, mouthwash, and many other products impacts the oral cavity. This may result in tooth decay, cavities, yellowish teeth, plaque building, and gum infections, which need effective prevention and treatment. However, due to a lack of financial resources, it becomes challenging for one to opt for the best and most effective service that can improve oral health conditions.

Inevitable Chronic Diseases

Poor oral health leads to various unavoidable chronic illnesses. Similarly, many chronic conditions can also aggravate oral diseases and infections. Inevitable chronic diseases like diabetes, HIV/AIDS, oral cancer, and many more are linked with increasing the chances of poor oral health. For instance, diabetic patients have lower resistance to infections, which leads to increased gum infections. The high sugar level in the blood often increases the sugar level in saliva. This high sugar in the saliva becomes the food for the bacteria residing in the plaque, which causes cavities, tooth decay, and gum diseases like gingivitis.

Apart from this, HIV/AIDS also impacts the immune function, which makes the body prone to oral infection and other severe illnesses. Patients with HIV/AIDS suffer from many oral problems like dry mouth, canker sores, tooth decay, and bone loss in the teeth during periodontitis. Further, osteoporosis not only impacts the bones in various parts of the body, but it can also reduce the jawbone density, which increases the risk of tooth loss. Similarly, many other chronic conditions like several types of cancers, rheumatoid arthritis, eating disorders, and immune system disorders also cause dry mouth, which can lead to many other oral health conditions, including gingivitis, dental caries, tooth enamel erosion, and halitosis.

Inability to Maintain Hygiene

Often, in a busy and hectic life schedule, one gets highly preoccupied with accomplishing their life goals, which often leads to an irresponsible attitude toward one's health. Numerous factors like lack of time, unawareness, and laziness often become the prime reason for ignoring basic hygiene habits like brushing teeth regularly, flossing teeth after every meal, cleaning the tongue, and swishing the mouth with mouthwash. The inability to maintain oral hygiene leads to plaque building, a colorless and sticky layer, which is the root cause of bacterial growth gum infections. All this eventually results in slowly damaging the teeth, gums, and oral cavity, which directly or indirectly has an unpleasant impact on the normal functioning of the body.

Poor or no oral hygiene is also the prime reason for bad breath and yellowish teeth that impact personality and confidence. Negligence toward maintaining good oral health also results in less frequent or no dental visits that refrain one from gaining an in-depth idea about their oral health problems and failure to recognize the early signs and symptoms, eventually leading to severe dental issues, thereby deteriorating one's overall health. Thus, one should be very mindful of following good and healthy hygiene habits and avoid skipping any of the oral health care regimes to ensure a long-lasting and bright smile.

Pica Disorder

One of the rare oral health conditions that arise due to lack of iron is also referred to as anemia in people. Due to pica disorder, the anemic person puts erosive and abrasive substances into their mouth, which has harsh impacts on the teeth and gum health. Pica disorder can have many severe and life-threatening impacts, but ones related to oral health are tooth decay, oral injuries like chipping teeth, abstraction, and abrasion. Individuals suffering from pica disorder crave to chew unhealthy items like cement, raw rice, chalk, ice, and raw clay. Eating and chewing such items, in the long run, will surely damage the gum and teeth enamel, which ends up in broken and damaged teeth.

Moreover, it is also responsible for disrupting the overall health of an individual by resulting in various unexpected diseases and problems. Pica disorder is often misconceived as an eating disorder or psychological disorder, but its impact on one's oral and overall health is irreversible. Once diagnosed with the symptoms of pica disorder, one must immediately visit a dentist to get a proper dental checkup done to prevent further deterioration of the teeth and gums and ensure the maintenance of the damaged ones.

Dental Trauma

Many times, despite having healthy and strong teeth, certain unfortunate circumstances like accidents or injuries often result in serious dental trauma that contributes to physical as well as mental stress. Any such dental accident that occurs in childhood is not a matter of concern as strong permanent teeth replace the milk teeth at a given time. However, when an adult encounters any such traumatic dental experience, the situation becomes more complicated as the damaged teeth need immediate attention and care. Various dental procedures like root canal treatment, tooth extraction, and denture replacements are required to retain a proper jawline and a perfect smile.

Apart from this, the physical discomfort and the special care that are required to maintain the teeth after these treatments serve as a barrier to achieving good oral health. Dental trauma creates complications in maintaining good oral health because the victim of such dental accidents feels scared to brush their teeth normally and also demands special attention from the dentists very frequently, which is time-consuming and is not budget friendly. So, in such cases, one must keep calm and strive their best to maintain the traumatized teeth by following the given instructions by the dentist and including the basic oral hygiene habits in their daily routine.

Chapter 6:

Quick Tips on Improving

Oral Health

A beautiful smile starts with healthy teeth. — Common
Phrase

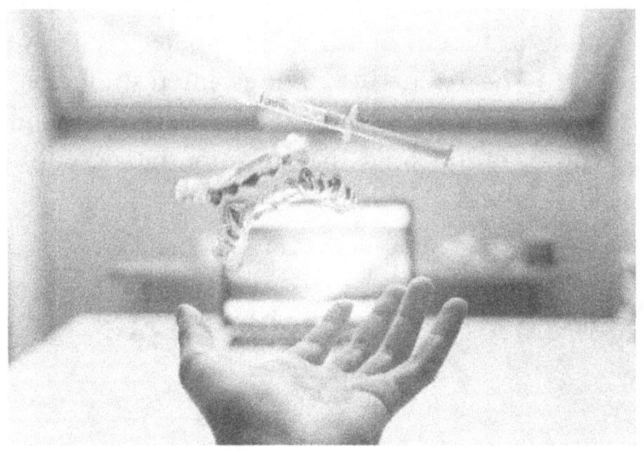

In a glamour-oriented world, where every individual
strives to create a unique identity and stand out in the
crowd, taking good care of one tooth, gums, and oral
health plays a crucial role. A healthy mouth not only
contributes toward one's strong personality, but it also
holds great importance for their overall wellness. As

truly said, the first impression is the last; a presentable smile defines a person's real personality.

In a world full of so many different people with varied ideologies, there are numerous good and bad pieces of advice that people may come up with, like brushing your teeth for not less than two to three minutes will give good results, using a non-fluoride toothpaste is a healthier option, flossing can create space between the teeth, and many more like this. However, embracing and following each one of them is not practically possible as different people have different situations and health conditions. But there are a few common must-dos for everyone that form the essential component of developing a healthy mouth by maintaining optimum oral hygiene. So, let's quickly dive deeper into the realms of various interesting tips and tricks that can help uncover the secrets of attaining a bright and beautiful smile, healthy mouth, and complete physical and mental wellness.

Brush Your Teeth Twice a Day

Improper teeth cleaning is often the most common factor that sows the seeds of oral health problems like bad breath, gum bleeding, toothache, and many more. Negligence to maintain oral hygiene impacts your smile by leaving the teeth yellowish and can become a breeding place for many harmful bacterial growth and infections. Brushing teeth twice a day is the recommended way to clean them after every meal, as it helps remove the food and dirt between the gums and teeth. However, the act of brushing improperly and in a poor way is of no use and is equivalent to not brushing teeth at all, as it can leave behind harmful bacteria and germs stuck in between the teeth and gums.

It is important to brush your teeth for two to three minutes and make sure to invest at least 30 seconds in each area, which helps in removing the harsh bacteria and preventing plaque formation. Spend good time cleaning the teeth every day by moving the brush in a circular motion that supports getting rid of the plaques, as hardened plaques are the foremost cause of calculus buildup, which results in mild tooth problems like gingivitis. Also, choosing a soft-bristled toothbrush instead of hard or medium bristles can prevent tooth enamel and gums from getting damaged. Always keep your toothbrush at a 45-degree angle toward the gums, as it helps remove the hard plaques and bacteria stuck at the gum line. Further, make it a habit to brush your teeth in all areas, including the sides, back, and front.

Clean Your Tongue

The tongue is the most neglected area in daily oral hygiene. Many of us are unaware of the fact that this often becomes the host to several diverse bacteria when we fail to pay proper attention. Plaque not only builds up on the teeth and gum line but can also accumulate on the tongue, as the tongue acts like a sponge to the bacteria. Plaque formation and bacteria on the tongue are the primary causes of bad breath and also initiate many other oral health problems. Further, an uncleaned tongue also limits its ability to taste the goodness of the food and refrains from getting the exact flavor. Apart from this, poor tongue hygiene also impacts digestive health and the immune system as it is the pathway for entering harmful bacteria and toxins into the body.

The simplest way to remove plaque and bacteria from the tongue layer is by using a soft bristle toothbrush or the tongue scraper. Open your mouth wide to stretch the tongue outside and start scraping from the middle of the tongue if you are a beginner. Place the scraper in the middle of the tongue and gently pull the stroke outward, scrape once or twice for one area. Make sure to wipe or wash off the scraper after each outward stroke to remove the debris from the surface. Repeat the process until you have cleaned the entire tongue. Apart from this, use anti-bacterial mouthwash every day to ensure that the oral cavity is free of any type of germs or bacteria. Alcohol-free mouthwash would reduce the chances of dry mouth and discomfort caused by it. Anti-bacterial mouthwash is an easy step to clean the tongue and teeth as it helps wash off the food debris and remove plaque build-up.

Use a Fluoride Toothpaste

Fluoride is a naturally occurring mineral that is found in many sources of food and drinking water. It is widely used as an important element of toothpaste as it is known for reducing the risk of tooth decay and gum infections. Fluoride is extensively popular for strengthening teeth and enamel by making it highly resistant to tooth decay, as it reduces the impact of acids produced by the bacteria accumulated in the plaques. Research claims that growing children with a high content of fluoride in their teeth have shallower grooves, which makes it easy to remove the plaque formed on the teeth. Although fluoride is found in water sources, toothpaste with this mineral helps protect the teeth from decay and infections. Children under the age of three must use toothpaste with a fluoride level of 1000 ppm. Children above three years of age and other adults must brush their teeth with toothpaste with a fluoride level of 1350 to 1500 ppm. However, in underdeveloped areas where the water supply does not have sufficient fluoride content, the tooth decay rate is much higher, up to five times more than that of the fluoridated area.

Fluoride can be added to the dental care routine in the form of toothpaste, mouthwash, and other supplements in order to prevent oral cavities and maintain good teeth health. In severe conditions where patients have serious cavities, the doctor prescribes mouthwash that contains a higher content of fluoride than in the other mouth products. Fluoride present in toothpaste and other oral health care products helps in rebuilding the weakened tooth enamel, reverses the signs of oral cavities and infections, reduces the growth of oral bacteria, and slows down demineralization from the tooth enamel. However, excessive use of fluoride can also have some side effects, majorly on children, if used in higher content in the form of toothpaste and drinking water, as it causes dental fluorosis. Dental fluorosis is a condition that causes white spots on the tooth surface, which eventually results in weakening and discoloration of the teeth.

Visit a Dentist Regularly

Maintaining good oral health is important not only to protect your teeth from several types of harmful oral diseases but also because it is responsible for overall health. There are two simple ways to build a healthy oral cavity: the preventive measures that prevent any gum disease from happening or the control measures that help in managing the symptoms and impacts of gum infections and diseases. In both cases, regular dental visits are a common step that combats the visible signs and impacts of tooth infection and gum diseases. Poor oral hygiene leads to plaque building on the teeth surface, which calcifies and takes the form of tartar. It is not easy to get rid of the tartar that accumulates on the teeth surface and becomes a breeding place for harmful bacteria and infections, eventually damaging gums and teeth. However, early action steps in the form of routine dentist checkups can help in avoiding such adverse situations and any further complications.

Regular dental visits are the key to making the patients feel accountable for their oral health. The dentist checks for the visible signs of infections and diseases and also analyses the regular habits that are responsible for causing them. During such visits, the dentist asks the patients about their eating habits, teeth grinding, smoking, and other addictive habits and risk factors that can cause gum diseases. Routine dental visits also ensure regular cleaning of teeth that helps in getting rid of the hard plaques and bacteria that can slowly damage the teeth and the gums. Apart from this, regular dentist checkups also help in deep cleaning the teeth of the patients who are suffering from mild gum infections. Patients with periodontal disease or other gum infections must also opt for regular dentist checkups as it helps extract information about the severity and progress of the problems that enables the dentist to make the apt decision for the patient's treatment plan.

Quit Tobacco and Alcohol

Smoking and alcohol are harmful to oral health as they cause adverse and irreversible situations that are difficult to cure. Addiction to alcohol and smoking both create an unhealthy oral environment that may deteriorate the teeth, enamel, and gums, causing tooth decay and cavities. Smoking directly impacts the immune system, which increases the chances of developing gum infections and diseases that are more difficult to treat. A smoker is at a higher risk of developing gum disease than a non-smoker. It is not easy for smokers to go through recovery therapies, as most of the efforts are ineffective. Regular smoking reduces the production of saliva in the mouth, causing dryness, and also impairs the functioning of the cells. Smoking increases the risk of many dental health problems like tooth decay, tooth loss, periodontal diseases, slow healing after treatment, discoloration of teeth, inflammation in the salivary glands, halitosis, plaque, and tartar buildup, and whitening of the soft tissues.

Consuming excess alcohol reduces the production of saliva, which causes dryness in the mouth. It is responsible for causing atrophy of the salivary glands that, in turn, interfere with the production of ADH (Adipic acid hydrazide), which regulates how much urine must be excreted by the body. When you consume alcohol in excess, the kidney tends to lose more water than normal, eventually dehydrating the body. Dehydration often causes a condition in most individuals called xerostomia or dry mouth. Research reveals that dry mouth is one of the major factors for developing several diseases like periodontitis (Zhu, 2022). Individuals consuming alcohol are at a greater risk of suffering from oral diseases, as it creates an acidic medium in the mouth, which leads to tooth erosion, tooth loss, oral cancer, tooth decay, receding gums, plaque building, and many more.

Don't Skip Flossing

Flossing is an important part of the oral hygiene routine. Ironically, it is often the most neglected part. Flossing daily before bedtime or after a meal helps ensure reduced or no cavities and gum diseases. Flossing is a key step in the dental hygiene routine that supports removing the food stuck between the teeth and prevents the formation of plaques. Sometimes, you may experience bleeding in the gums while flossing, which is a clear indication of any type of infection or gum disease. However, flossing daily helps to improve gum health by reducing gum bleeding over time. Flossing is crucial to good oral health not only because it helps in getting rid of the food particles stuck in between the teeth but also supports reducing plaques, stimulates the gums, and decreases the inflammation in that area. Further, it is also known for eliminating bad breath, reducing the risk of cavities, and preventing gingivitis, which can gradually progress into periodontal disease.

Limit the Intake of Sugars

Sugar consumption often seems harmless, but it can have adverse health implications for those who eat it. Eating a diet high in sugar often increases blood glucose levels, causing health issues like diabetes, obesity, heart disease, and early aging. However, the negative impacts of consuming a high-sugar diet are not limited to overall health. Unfortunately, it directly affects our oral health. Our mouth is a breeding place for many bacteria, some of which are beneficial while others are extremely harmful to oral health. According to research, some harmful bacteria produce large amounts of acids in the mouth when they come in contact with and digest sugar (Tan, 2017). These harmful acids are responsible for eroding the shiny protective layer on the teeth called enamel, a process called demineralization.

However, the saliva produced in the mouth acts as the constant healer that helps in reversing the damage caused by this process and is called remineralization. The minerals present in the saliva, like phosphate, calcium, and fluoride from the toothpaste, help in repairing the teeth' enamel by replacing it with the mineral that is lost due to the acid attacks of harmful bacteria, which strengthens the teeth. However, time and negligence to maintain good oral hygiene can lead to excessive mineral loss from the enamel and result in tooth decay and cavities. When the initial symptoms of tooth damage and cavities are left untreated, they seep into the deeper layers and result in pain, sensitivity, and tooth loss. Thus, consuming a diet that is less in sugar content can help in reducing the harsh impacts on the teeth.

Replace Your Old Toothbrush Often

We believe that taking care of oral health is a big responsibility that needs a strict routine of healthy habits and diet. However, we often fail to realize that maintaining good oral health is hidden in the small efforts that can bring about a miraculous change. Once you brush your teeth twice a day and maintain other hygiene habits, it is perceived that the teeth must stay healthy for life long. However, how long and when you must change the toothbrush is an overlooked topic that can cause great harm to dental health. Doctors recommend that it is a good habit to change a manual brush every three to five months (Stapleton, 2021). The bristles of the toothbrush become frayed and worn out after a few days of use, which must be replaced by another one as they lose their effectiveness.

Brushing teeth with an old toothbrush that has frayed bristles can miss out on cleaning the plaques and the debris stuck between the teeth, which increases the risk of tooth decay and cavities. Choosing the right toothbrush is an important factor that can assist in improving your oral health. Always place your toothbrush in a place where they don't come in contact with other toothbrushes. Wash and rinse the toothbrush after every use and place them vertically to let the bristles dry. Also, never keep the toothbrush in a closed container as it can lead to the growth of molds and bacteria, causing bacterial infection and various gum diseases.

Eat a Balanced Diet

A healthy mouth and good nutrition go hand in hand with each other. To achieve a healthy oral cavity, it is important to include a balanced diet from all the food groups that are rich in vitamins, minerals, calcium, and other beneficial substances that help in increasing teeth and gum health. Poor nutrition impacts the immune system, which reduces the resistance power of the body to fight against infection, which often contributes to periodontal disease. Research reveals that poor nutrition is not the exact cause of periodontal disease, but it is the major reason that leads to gum diseases and is faster in individuals with poor nutrition than the rest.

Apart from this, the food you eat comes in direct contact with the teeth and the teeth' enamel. Consuming a diet that is rich in sugary drinks, processed foods, and other items that are highly acidic can gradually erode the tooth enamel, which causes cavities and tooth decay. Thus, focusing on eating healthy food items and good nutrition can support accomplishing the goal of healthy oral health. Being mindful of eating habits is important not only for adults but also for teens and children because following an unhealthy diet from a very young age can cause tooth decay and cavities, especially if they follow poor oral hygiene habits. Some foods that must be avoided to maintain good oral health are sticky and starchy foods and snacks, acidic and sugary drinks, and soft drinks. Consuming foods like whole grains helps to provide magnesium, iron, and vitamin B, which keeps gum and teeth healthy. Eating fish, dairy products, eggs, and meat supplements with calcium and phosphorus are known for strengthening the bones and teeth and reducing the chances of tooth decay. Apart from this, including a diet rich in fruits, vegetables, fiber, protein, and healthy fats helps in making strong teeth and reduces inflammation, which improves overall oral health.

Chapter 7:

Mind-Boggling Facts

About Oral Health

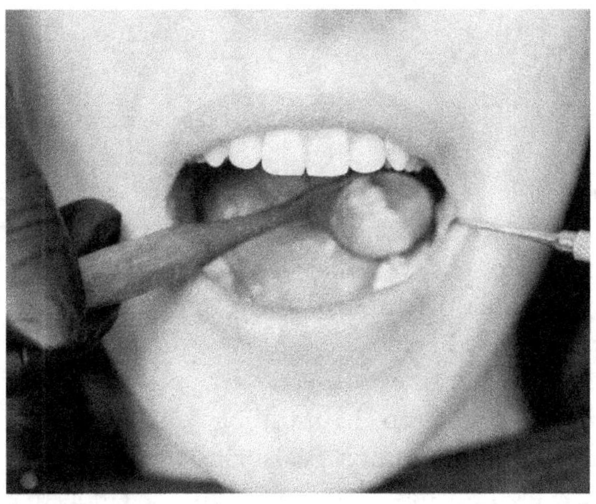

Brushing teeth daily to maintain a good mouth cavity
seems to be an everyday task and mundane affair that is
often taken for granted but less explored by many. The
world of dentistry is full of exciting stats and facts that
are truly astonishing. Nothing looks more appealing
than a bright, shining, and clean smile, as it is often the

first thing most people notice. Healthy teeth and gums are precious because they not only add outer beauty but also play a major role in boosting overall health. Despite being so important, most of the time, oral health has been neglected and less explored. But less known to many, the mouth cavity has a surplus of hidden amazing and exciting facts that can blow your mind and also support improved oral care. So, let's dig deeper and extract some of the most fascinating and entertaining facts about oral health that leave no room to surprise you.

Excess Chlorine Can Damage Tooth Enamel

Swimming is a great option for people who want to have fun and enjoy summer. However, staying back in the pool for hours can eventually take away your beautiful smile by the end of the summer, all due to a chemical called chlorine. At swimming pools and waterparks, chlorine is used extensively to help clean the water and keep harmful bacteria away. Adding chlorine to water supports balancing the pH level of the water, which kills away the unwanted bacteria that can cause harm. However, adding too much chlorine can lower the pH level, making the water acidic, which is not good for teeth health.

According to research, individuals who spend six hours or more per week in chlorinated water are at greater risk of facing unfavorable circumstances (Dental, 2022). Chlorinated water wears down the teeth' enamel, which increases sensitivity and tooth pain. Erosion of the protective enamel layer makes the teeth prone to decay and cavities. Apart from this, chlorinated water also leaves a stain on the teeth layer and causes dryness in the mouth. With consistent care, using fluoride toothpaste, managing the pH of the water, and reducing exposure to chlorine, one can reduce these harmful impacts. Also, avoid brushing your teeth soon after coming out of the swimming pool because chlorinated water softens the teeth' enamel for a short period, which can harm the teeth instead of doing good. Thus, be sure to brush your teeth after an hour or so to reduce the damage to tooth enamel.

Green Tea is Good for Healthy Gums

Green tea is famous among health-conscious people as it is a natural way of extracting many benefits for good health. Green tea is full of nutrients and multiple antioxidants, which help in reducing body fat, improving brain function, and lowering the risk of cancer naturally. Less known to many, green tea also serves amazing benefits for oral health. Research reveals that consuming green tea regularly helps improve teeth and gum health while lowering the chances of severe gum diseases like periodontitis (Goetz, 2023). Drinking one cup of green tea every day can help in reducing early tooth decay due to aging.

Green tea has natural antioxidant properties, which prevent the growth of bacteria, reduce plaque building, and lower the acidic content of saliva. Such characteristics of green tea help prevent cavities, oral infections, and gum diseases. Apart from this, green tea also helps in reducing bad breath from the mouth. Green tea has properties that kill the microbes in the mouth, which causes bad breath and makes one's mouth stinky. However, consuming excessive green tea can cause unwanted stains on the teeth with time. But with the right oral hygiene, these problems can be overcome easily to extract the other benefits for attaining healthier gums and teeth.

A Good Smile Boosts Immunity

A happy smile is a simple act that regular and impactful oral hygiene practices can achieve, but it is also known to serve miraculous benefits to one's lifestyle and overall health. One of the major requirements for attaining overall wellness is to have a good immune system functioning. Smiling not only makes one look confident and presentable but can also help boost immunity. When you smile, the body releases neurotransmitters that help to overcome the feeling of stress and anxiety and make you feel more relaxed. Strong immunity is an important aspect of a healthy life as it increases the resistance power of the body to fight against infection and diseases, which also boosts longevity.

A good smile not only adds beauty to the face but can also support reducing the signs of aging as it enhances the immune system. It is common to hear people say that smiling even in difficult situations is because it would heal the pain and make you feel better. A beautiful smile gifted by good oral hygiene and health is contagious and also supports adding beauty, positivity, and happiness in the lives of others, thus acting as a mood elevator. A smile not only shows confidence on the face when in social situations but also makes you look trustworthy and more approachable, which opens up the gate for improved social interaction and communication.

Tobacco and Smoking Causes Oral Cancer

Oral cancer is a serious medical condition that marks uncontrolled growth of the cancer cells in the mouth that convert into tumors. Oral cancer can occur anywhere in the mouth cavity, including the tongue, gums, cheeks, lips, floor, roof, and back of the mouth. Tobacco consumption is known to increase the risk of developing oral cancers as they are carcinogenic and can modify the genetics of the cells present in the oral cavity, which causes oral cancers. Tobacco use is directly linked with increasing the risk of oral cancers, as it exposes the mouth cavity to carcinogenic chemicals either by chewing or smoking tobacco products.

Tobacco is a harmful and addictive substance that is present in cigarettes, pipe tobacco, cigars, snuff, and chewing tobacco. Tobacco is comprised of nicotine that causes addiction, toxins that are poisonous substances, and carcinogens that cause cancers. Each tobacco product is dangerous to the oral cavity as excessive consumption is known to increase the risk of developing cancer at different places in the mouth. According to research, smokers are at ten times higher risk of developing oral cancer than non-smokers. Smoking cigars is considered to be less harmful than compared to cigarettes, as it avoids inhaling the harmful substances. However, cigars and pipe tobacco increase the chances of developing lip cancers, oral cancers, and cancer in other parts like the lungs, esophagus, and voice box. Apart from this, consuming tobacco in the form of chewing tobacco and snuff that is not directly inhaled also causes several types of cancers in the oral cavity, including gums, cheeks, and lips.

Flossing Teeth Increases Life Expectancy

Flossing is a crucial part of oral hygiene that helps maintain good teeth and gum health. Flossing also serves other benefits to the body that not only help reduce the chances of many chronic diseases but also improve life expectancy. Flossing is a simple process that prevents plaque building and keeps unwanted bacteria away from the teeth layer. Negligence to remove the plaques from the teeth results in the formation of hard deposits called tartar that cause irritation and inflammation. These symptoms eventually result in gum disease called periodontitis, which in many cases can be associated with many other ailments in the body, like diabetes, heart diseases, mouth cancers, kidney disorders, and Alzheimer's diseases.

Lack of flossing is not directly linked with causing any such disease, but the inflammation caused by this gum disease aggravates other severe conditions in the body, thereby creating a life-threatening situation. Thus, when dental health is concerned, one must be very mindful about following each step toward maintaining healthy hygiene habits, as well as eating habits that will eventually ensure one's overall wellness and a long life.

Brushing Cleans Only 60 Percent of Teeth

Lack of awareness and knowledge often supports the notion that brushing teeth alone is one of the best and sufficient ways to maintain a healthy mouth and teeth. However, the reality is far beyond one's imagination, as apart from brushing, various other essential oral hygiene habits help retain healthier teeth lifelong. Flossing teeth, using mouthwash, cleaning the tongue, and maintaining healthy eating habits are important practices that cannot be overlooked, even in the short run.

Simply brushing teeth contributes to cleaning three out of five teeth, which approximates to 60% of the cleaning process only, which is not sufficient enough to maintain a healthy and bright smile with strong, shiny teeth. Thus, it is a must for everyone to inculcate all the above-mentioned oral hygiene habits in one's daily routine religiously to get visible positive effects on oral and overall health.

Knocked Out Teeth Can be Fixed

Many times, due to accidents or while playing outdoor sports like baseball or football, one might encounter severe mouth injuries that can result in teeth damage. In the worst cases, these can even lead to the knocking down of teeth, which can be extremely painful due to the physical damage and bleeding. In such circumstances, it is obvious for anyone to panic and feel scared as it calls for an emergency. However, due to unawareness and negligence of people, it may become impossible to restore the broken teeth as they might discard them or not take the proper required action.

In the case of adults, the knocked-out teeth can be restored by immediately placing the teeth back in their original position before one seeks medical assistance. Once the tooth is placed in its right place, the chances of its survival increase. However, in the case of kids who have primary teeth, any knocked-out teeth must not be placed back in the mouth as it may cause damage to the permanent teeth developing beneath the gums. Moreover, one should never try to skip seeking a dentist's advice in case of any such teeth trauma, as it may hinder the restoration process of the teeth. Thus, with immense patience, one should immediately provide the necessary first aid before seeking the doctor, which can be an appropriate effort toward retaining one's teeth and overall health.

Our Teeth are Stronger Than Our Bones

Hardly any of us may know a surprising fact about teeth. They have the hardest structure in the body, called enamel. It is difficult to believe that tooth enamel is much stronger than bones. In our daily lives, most of us often experience chipping of teeth, while bone breaking is a rare instance. Our tooth enamel is densely packed with various minerals, making our teeth strong and durable. Both tooth enamel and bones are made up of the same mineral called hydroxyapatite, which is a naturally occurring mineral similar to calcium apatite. Calcium is an important component needed by the bones and the teeth to retain their strength.

Although bones and teeth are comprised of the same mineral, still tooth enamel is harder than the bones because it has a greater content of hydroxyapatite. Bones are made up of 70% hydroxyapatite, while the tooth enamel contains around 96%, which makes it the hardest of all. However, the greater hardness of the tooth enamel makes it more brittle, which is the prime reason it gets chipped off more easily than compared with the bones. Tooth enamel is hard, but they are also more brittle, which makes it necessary for one to take excessive care to prevent damage and chipping off due to unhealthy eating habits, poor oral hygiene, and teeth accidents.

Chapter 8:

Bust the Myths About Oral Health and Hygiene

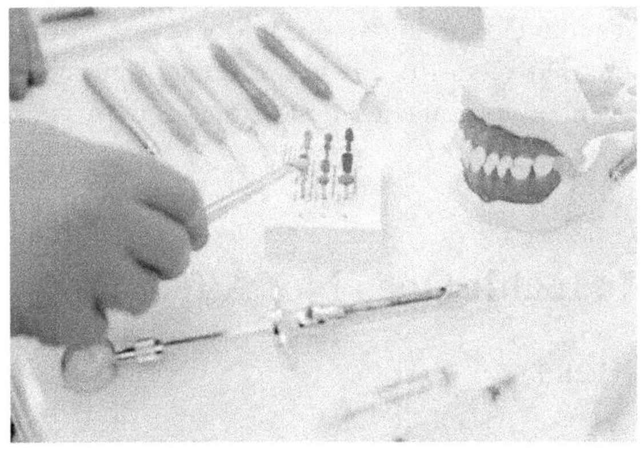

A beautiful smile is a great blessing, which is not possible without healthy gums and bright teeth. However, owning this smile and maintaining it is a big challenging task, as in the current era where we have a stock of various alluring options to feast upon, like junk food, beverages, and desserts; it is not possible to stay away from dental issues. We live in a social world, where every problem or issue is presented and perceived in numerous ways, thus giving rise to multifarious thoughts and ideas about any particular context. This, on the other hand, gives rise to inappropriate beliefs and misconceptions that hover in the minds of the people, making them prey to the false notions set by the crowd. Many a time, these heard-and-said fallacies are just irrelevant talk of the town and have no significance in reality. Unfortunately, as these myths circulate around us, they make space in our minds, and we start believing them blindly, thereby influencing our lives and health on the whole. Thus, it is important for us to explore and understand the reality behind such ideologies in order to create awareness among the people and make them well-equipped with the basics of maintaining good oral and overall health. So, let's unveil the most common myths about oral health and hygiene to create awareness among people to prevent any dental complications and problems in the future.

Oral Health Does Not Affect Overall Wellness

One of the biggest misconceptions that most of us often fall prey to is that oral health and overall health are two different aspects that have no interrelationship with each other. Due to unawareness and irresponsible attitude toward oneself, people fall prey to many different unexpected diseases and health issues that are not directly related to any type of oral or dental problem. However, on visiting a dentist or consulting experts, one can easily understand that oral health forms an intact part of one's complete wellness. Thus, one must be very careful and active while caring for their teeth and oral cavity. It will support good overall health by improving immunity and increasing lifespan.

Cutting off Sugar Prevents Cavities

Consuming sugar is often considered to be one of the biggest reasons for increasing cavities in people nowadays. However, scientific evidence does not support this, and thus, weird myths like this are created, which tend to mislead us. It is true that eating sugar or sugary food items supports the growth of unhealthy bacteria in our mouths as it becomes their food. However, completely cutting off sugar from the diet does not ensure a healthy mouth, as many different food items serve as a source of sugar and its compounds in our diet. Many times, we overlook the fact that the main reason behind the building up of cavities in our mouth is the stuck food particles and debris that need not be rich in sugar specifically. Accumulation of food particles in our teeth and oral cavity creates a bacteria-friendly atmosphere in our mouth that helps in the growth and survival of harmful bacteria within our mouth, thereby encouraging tooth damage and cavities. Thus, maintaining a healthy mouth with strong teeth and gums does not only depend on what we eat; instead, it is governed by the way we follow and maintain the basic oral hygiene habits in our lives. So, one must always follow basic oral hygiene practices like brushing one's teeth twice a day, flossing teeth after eating anything, and refreshing mouth using effective mouthwash.

Aging Does Not Deteriorate Teeth Health

Aging is a natural phenomenon that causes various changes in the cells, tissues, and other organs of our body, including our teeth. As one ages, the process of wear and tear starts, which can be even seen in one's oral health, like the formation of gaps between the teeth, loosening and decolorizing of teeth, and many such visible symptoms. Old age causes various health disorders that compel one to rely on medicines to keep them healthy. This, in turn, impacts oral health, as the secretion of saliva is reduced, which results in a dry mouth. Furthermore, dryness in the mouth triggers the growth of harmful bacteria, causing plaque and cavities. Thus, aging has a negative impact on the oral health of an individual, resulting in many dental problems. So, with growing age, one should take special care to retain the life of their teeth and maintain a healthy mouth.

All Tooth Fillings Are Safe

When we visit a dentist to repair damaged teeth, the dentist often uses fillings to save the teeth by preventing any plaque and bacterial buildup in the broken or cracked teeth. These fillings are available in various different types like amalgam filling, composite filling, and porcelain filling. Due to a lack of basic knowledge about dental procedures, many assume that all these dental fillings are safe for us. However, the fact is far different from this as only porcelain fillings are a safer and non-toxic way of restoring damaged teeth. On the other hand, amalgam fillings have mercury in them, which releases toxic vapors when used over the long run and causes various health issues like allergic reactions, multiple sclerosis, oral cancer, and thyroid disorders. Moreover, the composite filling also has harmful substances, like BPA, BHT, etc., that are toxic to the human body. Despite knowing the disadvantages of such harmful fillings, people still go for them as they are a cheaper option as compared to porcelain filling. So, before you get your teeth mended by some sort of filling, explore and know the pros and cons of each one of them to be responsible for any unexpected health complication in the future.

Dental X-rays are Life-Threatening

Dental X-rays are one of the important procedures that the dentist performs in order to figure out any problem beneath the gums and roots of the teeth, which cannot be easily diagnosed with the naked eye. It is normal to get an X-ray done when you visit a dentist during a routine cleaning and check-up session. The main concern behind the concept of dental X-rays is that they use radiation to diagnose issues related to the teeth. Most people often believe that undergoing dental X-rays exposes them to this harmful radiation that can cause cancer, which can even be life-threatening. However, the fact contradicts this as research reveals that dental X-rays are completely safe for monitoring one's oral health when performed using minimal radiation and in moderation. Moreover, all possible measures are taken by the dentist to ensure the safety of the patients while performing dental X-rays like the use of lead aprons and leaded thyroid collars. However, performing dental X-rays on young children, old people, and pregnant women is an arguable issue as they are vulnerable and easily susceptible to radiation damage. So, one should have complete knowledge and awareness about the right way to get the dental X-ray done within the right time span to prevent any sort of health complications.

Smoking Only Decolorizes Teeth

In today's world, when the unhealthy habit of addiction is becoming very common among people, smoking cigarettes and cigars has become a rising trend. People are increasingly embracing this injurious habit without even pondering over the harmful drawbacks that it can have on one's overall health. Many of us often think that smoking simply deteriorates our oral health by decolorizing teeth and damaging the oral cavity. However, the fact is far more dreadful than this, as smoking mainly damages the lungs and the respiratory system on the whole, which eventually impacts the immunity and lifespan of an individual negatively. In the worst situation, smoking leads to oral cancer, lung cancer, and other such life-threatening diseases that can leave a profound scar on one's mind and life. So, one must wisely consider the pros and cons of everything that is related to one's oral health, as it can help them make the best decision for the betterment of their overall health.

Chapter 9:

Healthy Mouth: A Window

to Assess Your Sane Body

Don't let dental problems creep up on you; be proactive in taking care of your oral health. —Common Phrase

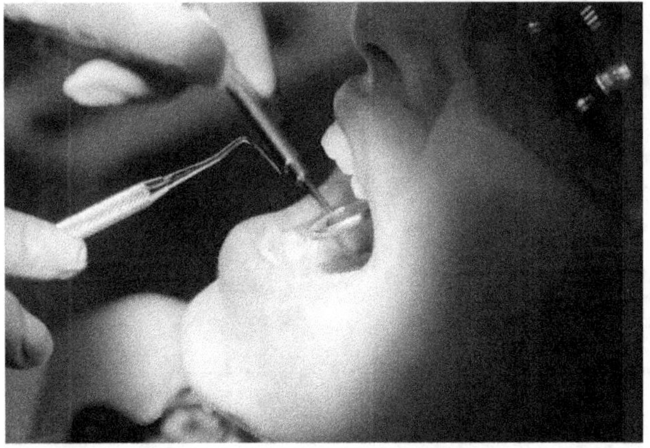

Many a time, people fail to understand the importance of maintaining good oral hygiene, which unfortunately takes them in a direction that disturbs their lifestyle in a negative manner. Moreover, in the busy chaos of life where everyone is rushing to achieve their goals and targets, people hardly get time to visit a dentist to ensure proper care and health of their mouth. Due to all these unexplained factors, various unanswered questions remain neglected, which are a red flag for some major health issues cropping up in the future. So, here we are with an interesting set of self-evaluation questions that will surely assist you in knowing your oral health condition and will also help you keep a number of illnesses and diseases at bay, thereby improving the overall quality of your life.

Evaluate Your Oral Health

How many times do you brush your teeth in a day?

1. Once

2. Twice

3. Thrice

4. None of the Above

What type of toothbrush do you use?

1. Hard bristles

2. Soft bristles

3. Electric toothbrush

4. Not using a toothbrush

What type of toothpaste do you use?

1. Fluoridated Toothpaste

2. Herbal Toothpaste

3. Sensitivity Toothpaste

4. None of the Above

How often do you visit a dentist?

1. Once a Month

2. Once in 6 Months

3. Once a Year

4. Never

What do you use to floss your teeth?

1. Toothpick

2. Waxed String Floss

3. Unwaxed String Floss

4. Nothing

How often do you floss your teeth?

1. Daily

2. Once a Week

3. After Every Meal

4. Never

How often do you change your toothbrush?

1. Once in 3 Months

2. Once in 6 Months

3. Once a Year

4. Never

How frequently do you use mouthwash?

1. Daily

2. Once a Month

3. Once in 6 Months

4. Never

For how long should you swish your teeth with mouthwash?

1. 10 seconds

2. 30 seconds

3. 1 minute

4. 2 minutes

How do you whiten your teeth?

1. Professional Teeth Whitening by Dentist

2. Homemade Hacks to Whiten Your Teeth

3. Teeth Whitening Toothpaste

4. None of the Above

Think and Answer

Does your diet contain more sugar or acidic food?

1. Yes

2. No

Do you have plaque buildup on your teeth?

1. Yes

2. No

Does your mouth smell or do you have bad breath?

1. Yes

2. No

Are your teeth discolored?

1. Yes

2. No

Do you have cavities in your teeth?

1. Yes

2. No

Do you experience any tooth or gum pain?

1. Yes

2. No

Do you suffer from any of the chronic disorders?

1. Yes

2. No

Do you visit a dentist regularly?

1. Yes

2. No

Do you smoke or consume tobacco products?

1. Yes

2. No

Do you consume excess caffeinated products?

1. Yes

---

2. No

Do you feel tooth sensitivity while eating and drinking?

1. Yes

2. No

Do you need cosmetic treatment to improve your smile?

1. Yes

2. No

Do you use an electric toothbrush?

1. Yes

2. No

Do you brush your teeth before going to bed?

1. Yes

2. No

Do you floss your teeth?

1. Yes

2. No

Do you use mouthwash after brushing and flossing your teeth?

1. Yes

2. No

Do you use natural mouth deodorizer to prevent bad breath?

1. Yes

2. No

Do you use a tongue scraper to clean your tongue?

1. Yes

2. No

Do you use teeth whitening products?

---

1. Yes

2. No

Do you have a bad habit of tooth grinding?

1. Yes

2. No

Do you know the red flags of unhealthy oral health?

1. Yes

2. No

Do you maintain basic oral hygiene?

1. Yes

2. No

Do you eat a balanced diet rich in calcium and vitamin D?

1. Yes

2. No

Do you have loose teeth?

1. Yes

2. No

Have you ever been embarrassed due to oral health issues?

1. Yes

2. No

Are you satisfied with your oral and overall health?

1. Yes

2. No

Conclusion

Easy Steps to Get a Sane Body Through a Healthy Mouth is an interesting guide to winning millions of hearts with a bright smile by *Karah Viniz*. The book is the best read for all health and image-conscious people who wish to make a big difference in their lives with a healthy mouth and strong teeth. The book introduces the readers to the basics of maintaining oral hygiene by finding genuine answers to interesting questions about dental health. It also highlights the essential must-haves that every individual should own in order to achieve a presentable and beautiful smile. Moreover, the book throws light on the life-changing benefits of having good oral health that directly or indirectly have a drastic impact on the overall wellness of an individual as well.

Apart from this, the book aims to forewarn the readers by highlighting the red flags that serve as a prior indication of any approaching dental issue. As we move ahead, the book presents the most common risk factors that aggravate one's oral and overall health. The book will also discuss the major barriers that may come in the way of attaining a healthy mouth and sane body. It also equips the readers with simple and practical tips and advice that can help one ease the journey toward developing oral hygiene habits that will serve as an eye-opener for the readers. Furthermore, the book is a perfect blend of various mind-boggling facts and interesting myths that will surely keep the readers entertained with its uniqueness. The book also provides an elaborate worksheet that will help the readers access their oral as well as overall health.

Lastly, I would like to convey my hearty thanks to all the passionate readers who dedicated their precious time to reading the book and understanding its purpose. I would be very happy and excited to read your reviews for the book, as your feedback is valuable to me and can guide me to create more relatable and interesting content like this. So, before you turn back the pages of the book, let's think over a few engaging questions that might be hovering in your head by now:

- Do I have a healthy mouth?

- Does my oral health impact my overall health?

- Do I have symptoms of poor oral health?

- Should I visit a dentist more frequently?

- Do I have any misconceptions about my oral health?

- How can I ease my journey toward achieving a healthy mouth and a sane body?

Glossary

Alzheimer's Disease: A brain disease that gets worse with time and is similar to dementia, which generally triggers during old age, causing memory loss, disorientation, impaired thinking, and drastic changes in personality.

Antidepressants: A type of drugs or medications that are used for getting relief from depression.

Antihistamines: A kind of compound that counteracts the histamine in the body and is used to treat various allergic conditions.

Auto-Immune Diseases: A type of disease in which the body's immune system attacks the healthy cells of the body.

Carcinogenic: Anything that tends to cause cancer.

Celiac Diseases: A hereditary intestinal disorder in which they lose the ability to absorb gliadin, which eventually damages intestinal mucosa.

Decongestants: A medicine that relieves congestion.

Demineralization: A medical condition in which the body loses the minerals.

Dentures: A set of artificial teeth that replace the real ones.

Diuretics: A type of medicine that reduces the build-up of fluid in the body.

Halitosis: An oral health condition in which a person has a foul-smelling mouth.

Hypertension: A health condition in which a person has high blood pressure.

Microbiome: A community of different microorganisms that live together in a habitat.

Orofacial: Anything related to face and mouth.

Socially Disadvantaged: A group of individuals subjected to prejudice and bias.

World Health Organization: A special agency of the United Nations that deals with issues related to international public health.

References

Archibald, J. (2020, December 6). *Bad breath (Halitosis)*. Healthline. https://www.healthline.com/health/bad-breath#diagnosis

Author. (2023, July 18). *Dental quotes for patients*. Fsmstatistics.fm. https://fsmstatistics.fm/dental-quotes-for-patients/#:~:text=%E2%80%9CYour%20smile%20is%20your%20greatest

Cafasso, J. (2014, November 6). *Everything you need to know about dental and oral health*. Healthline. https://www.healthline.com/health/dental-and-oral-health

Cherney, K. (2015a, August 20). *11 Best practices for healthy teeth*. Healthline. https://www.healthline.com/health/dental-and-oral-health/best-practices-for-healthy-teeth#Take-care-of-your-teeth

Cherney, K. (2015b, August 20). *11 Ways to Keep Your Teeth Healthy*. Healthline; Healthline Media. https://www.healthline.com/health/dental-and-oral-health/best-practices-for-healthy-teeth

Compton, K. (2023, September 5). *Oral health: Its importance in comprehensive health care.*

Drugwatch.com.
https://www.drugwatch.com/health/oral-health/

Dental, S. (2022, June 16). *Can pool chlorine damage your teeth?* Sunrise Dental. https://sunrisedentalarizona.com/can-pool-chlorine-damage-your-teeth/#:~:text=However%2C%20if%20there

Dr. Micheal. (2018, April 7). *53 best dental quotes to brighten your smile!* Dr. Michaels Dental Clinic. https://www.drmichaels.com/blog/best-dental-quotes

Everett, D. J. (2022, November 7). *How bad oral hygiene can lead to oral cancer.* Kirkland Dental. https://kirklandteeth.com/general-dentistry/bad-oral-hygiene-oral-cancer/

Frank, C. (2014, November 6). *Preventing oral health problems.* Healthline. https://www.healthline.com/health/dental-oral-health-prevention

Frank, C. (2019, March 14). *The 8 best practice healthy teeth and gums.* Medical News Today. https://www.medicalnewstoday.com/articles/324708

Goetz, N. (2023, January 26). *Prevent gum disease naturally: Drink green tea regularly.* Ocean Breeze Prosthodontics. https://oceanbreezeprosthodontics.com/general/prevent-gum-disease-naturally/#:~:text=Because%20green%20tea%20controls%20bacteria

Gotter, A. (2018, February 9). *Sensitive teeth: Causes, symptoms, treatments, and more.* Healthline. https://www.healthline.com/health/sensitive-teeth#What-causes-sensitive-teeth?

Higuera, V. (2017, October 18). *Loose teeth in adults: What you should know.* Healthline; Healthline Media. https://www.healthline.com/health/loose-tooth

Imai, K., Iinuma, T., & Sato, S. (2021). Relationship between the oral cavity and respiratory diseases: Aspiration of oral bacteria possibly contributes to the progression of lower airway inflammation. *Japanese Dental Science Review, 57,* 224–230. https://doi.org/10.1016/j.jdsr.2021.10.003

Jovinally, J. (2015, June 2). *Type 2 diabetes and oral health.* Healthline. https://www.healthline.com/health/type-2-diabetes/oral-health#risk-factors

Mark, A. M. (2016). Diabetes and oral health. *The Journal of the American Dental Association, 147*(10), 852. https://doi.org/10.1016/j.adaj.2016.07.010

Parker, H. (2022, April 22). *The basics of gum problems.* WebMD. https://www.webmd.com/oral-health/gum-problem-basics-sore-swollen-and-bleeding-gums

Sahi, A. (2020, September 16). *What microorganisms naturally live in the mouth?* News-Medical. https://www.news-medical.net/health/What-Microorganisms-Naturally-Live-in-the-Mouth.aspx

Song, A. (2019, December 20). *11 Dental myths and misconceptions.* 209 NYC Dental. https://www.209nycdental.com/11-dental-myths-and-misconceptions/

Stanborough, R. J. (2019, August 2). *Dental plaque : What it Is, what causes It, and how to get rid of I.* Healthline. https://www.healthline.com/health/dental-and-oral-health/plaque#treatment

Stapleton, M. (2021, January 6). *How often should you change your toothbrush.* Chaska Dentist Blog. https://www.chaskadentist.com/blog/2021/01/06/how-often-should-you-change-your-toothbrush/#:~:text=According%20to%20the%20Centers%20for

Tan, V. (2017, April 6). *How sugar causes cavities and destroys your teeth.* Healthline. https://www.healthline.com/nutrition/how-sugar-destroys-teeth#TOC_TITLE_HDR_3

University of Illinois Chicago. (2019, August 19). *The many costs (Financial and Well-Being) of poor oral health | College of Dentistry | University of Illinois Chicago.* Dentistry. https://dentistry.uic.edu/news-stories/the-many-costs-financial-and-well-being-of-poor-

oral-
health/#:~:text=Financial%20limitations%20of
ten%20prevent%20people

Williams, A. (2022, April 20). *What you need to know about mouth ulcers.* Healthline. https://www.healthline.com/health/mouth-ulcers#prevention-tips

World Health Organization. (2022a). *Cardiovascular diseases.* World Health Organization. https://www.who.int/health-topics/cardiovascular-diseases#tab=tab_1

World Health Organization. (2022b, November 18). *Oral health.* Who.int; World Health Organization: WHO. https://www.who.int/news-room/fact-sheets/detail/oral-health

World Health Organization. (2023). *Oral health.* Oral Health. https://www.who.int/health-topics/oral-health#tab=tab_1

Zhu, D. C. (2022, April 12). *Effects of alcohol and smoking on oral health.* Freedom Dental. https://www.dentistinfairfield.com/effects-of-alcohol-and-smoking-on-oral-health/#:~:text=Alcohol%20and%20smoking%20are%20harmful

Image Reference

Babydov, I. (2021, May 5). *Human skull holding toothbrush between teeth* *[Online Image]*. Pexels. https://www.pexels.com/photo/human-skull-holding-toothbrush-between-teeth-7787979/

Diamond, S. (2020, February 18). *Woman with red lipstick smiling* *[Online Image]*. Pexels. https://www.pexels.com/photo/woman-with-red-lipstick-smiling-3762453/

Fauntleroy, C. (2020a, April 29). *An open mouth of a person* *[Online Image]*. Pexels. https://www.pexels.com/photo/an-open-mouth-of-a-person-4269690/

Fauntleroy, C. (2020b, April 29). *Crop unrecognizable stomatologist with tweezers and dental tools in clinic* *[Online Image]*. Pexels. https://www.pexels.com/photo/crop-unrecognizable-stomatologist-with-tweezers-and-dental-tools-in-clinic-4269362/

Frank, D. (2017, February 4). *Syringe floating near person's hand* *[Online Image]*. Pexels. https://www.pexels.com/photo/syringe-floating-near-person-s-hand-287227/

Isil. (2023, February 23). *Toothbrush, a tube of toothpaste and a smile painted with toothpaste [Online Image].* Pexels. https://www.pexels.com/photo/toothbrush-a-a-tube-of-toothpaste-and-a-smile-painted-with-toothpaste-15694640/

Lane, A. (2020, November 20). *Smile made of ripe fruits [Online Image]*. Pexels. https://www.pexels.com/photo/smile-made-of-ripe-fruits-5946078/

Philomin, A. (2022, May 15). *Dentist checking teeth of a person [Online Image]*. Pexels. https://www.pexels.com/photo/dentist-checking-teeth-of-a-person-12148417/

Piacquadia, A. (2020, February 20). *Dentist working on woman's teeth [Online Image]*. Pexels. https://www.pexels.com/photo/dentist-working-working-on-woman-s-teeth-3779713/

www.ingramcontent.com/pod-product-compliance
Lightning Source LLC
Chambersburg PA
CBHW072240150726
48002CB00005B/2179